Contents

NURSING RESEARCH
Setting new agendas

WITH

Edited by

Pam Smith PhD, MSc, BNurs, DNCert, HV Cert,
Cert Ed, RNT
Professor of Nursing, Redwood College of Health Studies,
South Bank University, London

A member of the Hodder Headline Group
LONDON • NEW YORK • SYDNEY • AUCKLAND

First published in Great Britain in 1998 by
Arnold, a member of the Hodder Headline Group
338 Euston Road, London NW1 3BH
http://www.arnoldpublishers.com

British Library Cataloguing in Publication Data
A catalogue record for this book is available from the British Library

Library of Congress Cataloging-in-Publication Data
A catalog record for this book is available from the Library of Congress

ISBN 0 340 66194 1

Commissioning Editor: Clare Parker
Production Editor: James Rabson
Production Controller: Priya Gohil
Cover designer: Terry Griffiths

Composition in 10/12pt Palatino by Photoprint, Torquay, Devon
Printed and bound in Great Britain by J W Arrowsmith Ltd, Bristol

List of contributors

Olwyn Bamford RGN, DipN, BSc (Hons)
Senior Nurse
Practice Development
University College London Hospital Trust
London

Gosia Brykczyńska BA, BSc, CertEd, DipPH, RGN/RSCN, RNT,
    Onc. Cert
Lecturer in Ethics and Philosophy
Royal College of Nursing Institute
London

Angie Cotter PhD, Dip Health Ed, BSc (SocSci), RN
Senior Research Fellow
City University St Bartholomew's School of Nursing and
    Midwifery
Honorary Senior Research Fellow, Kings Healthcare Trust
London

Trudi James RGN, BSc(Hons), Dip HV, MSc
Research Fellow
School of Health and Social Care
South Bank University
London

Anne Jones RGN, MSc
Associate Researcher
Department of Nursing Studies
King's College
University of London
London

Maureen E. Lahiff MSc, RN, RM, BTA Cert, HV, CHNT
Independent Consultant
formerly: Professor of Nursing
CNA Bloomsbury Health Authority
Adviser/Lecturer in Management and Leadership
Royal College of Nursing

Maria Lorentzon PhD, MSc(Soc), RN, RM
Honorary Research Fellow in General Practice
Imperial College School of Medicine at St Mary's
London

Helen Mann RGN, ENB 870 (Research)
Clinical Nurse Specialist
St George's Hospital
London

Abigail Masterson MN, BSc, RGN, PGCEA
Director
International Nursing Ltd
Bristol

Pam Smith PhD, MSc, BNurs, RGN, DNCert, HV Cert, Cert Ed,
    RNT
Professor of Nursing
Redwood College of Health Studies
South Bank University
London

Colleen Wedderburn Tate MSc, BA, DMS, Cert Ed, RN, RM,
    Fellow RSA
Independent Nurse Researcher
Presiden
CWT Enterprises

Dawn Whittaker BA, RGN, MSc
Health Advisor
Ambrose King Centre
The Royal London Hospital
London

1

Setting the nursing research agenda: topics, approaches and methods

Pam Smith

In this chapter the editor introduces the book and sets the scene for the ensuing chapters. The rationale behind the book, the choice of topics and authors and the production process are described. The authors were invited to contribute to the book because of their experience and expertise in particular fields. Subsequently, each chapter provides an opportunity for them to explore the issues associated with their field as a means for influencing nursing's research agenda.

Introduction

A recent perusal of the nursing research texts available in a leading university bookshop, by the editor, Pam Smith, revealed a complete aisle dedicated to the topic. This experience led to two questions. First, why were there so many texts committed to research in a specific discipline compared with, say, the medical and engineering shelves? Second, given there were so many books currently available, was there indeed a need for yet another one?

In answer to the first question we can speculate that as relative new-comers to the world of academe and research, nurses have begun to build both their self-confidence and research culture through authorship. The majority of the book titles and contents represented different approaches to doing research. Books dedicated to the presentation of research findings were less in evidence. As Maureen Lahiff informs us in Chapter 3, many of the early nursing research studies were unsuccessful in finding commercial publishers. Nursing research was clearly not considered of sufficient inter-est to attract a viable readership nor to merit the financial risk involved in wide dissemination. Early exceptions included Charlotte Kratz's (1978) investigation into the community care of the long-term sick and an edited collection of research studies on patient and midwifery care (Wilson-Barnett, 1983).

Our answer to the second question as to whether yet another research textbook is required, is a definite 'yes'. Our book is different because it serves as a bridge between books about the processes of research and books about its findings. Our purpose is to assist the reader to ask questions in order to get behind the assumptions on which the theory and practice of research in general and nursing research in particular are based. These questions are designed to examine and challenge the nature and origins of research and the different philosophical and methodological approaches used to study nursing and health care.

Of particular importance to a book which aims to get behind research assumptions are questions about the pre-investigation phase of ideas and agendas. Where do ideas come from and who sets the research agenda? Which factors shape that agenda and whose interests do they serve? How does a topic get selected as a suitable subject for study? Which factors influence the adoption of particular research approaches? How useful is it to make the distinction between qualitative and quantitative research?

Other questions follow about the primary purpose of research. Is it to maintain the *status quo* within society or does it have the potential to liberate groups who are traditionally marginalized because of their race, gender, class, sexual orientation, occupation or lack of it? If, as Abigail Masterson suggests in Chapter 5, nursing is a marginalized occupation, how can frontline practitioners influence the research agenda and what use does research have for them? Furthermore, what is the relationship between research, knowledge and practice? How does research generate new knowledge and how can it be used to evaluate practice? What impact has the 'contract culture' had on research and practice?

In our quest to seek answers, we refer to the work of Paul Feyerabend, described by Gosia Brykczyńska in Chapter 6 as the *enfant terrible* of the philosophy of science.

Feyerabend wrote in 1978:

> There is no 'scientific method'; there is no single procedure, or set of rules that underlies every piece of research and guarantees that it is 'scientific' and therefore trustworthy. Every project, every theory, every procedure has to be judged on its own merits and by standards adapted to the processes with which it deals. The idea of a universal and stable *method* that is an unchanging measure of adequacy and even the idea of a universal and stable *rationality* is as unrealistic as the idea of a universal and stable measuring instrument that measures any magnitude, no matter what the circumstances. (p. 98)

Feyerabend's statement invites us to seek new ways of seeing and being involved in research. He also helps us to address one of the central preoccupations of nursing research about drawing distinctions between qualitative and quantitative research. Colleen Wedderburn Tate's Chapter 2 explores further some of the issues about the certainty of scientific theory and method and challenges its singular appropriateness to the study of nursing and health care.

We also incorporate the view of sociologist, C. Wright Mills (1970), who argued that in order to study society it is necessary to see each individual as a minute intersection of biography and history. Only then can researchers understand what is happening in the world and to individuals. The intersection of biography with history is a powerful place. Each chapter demonstrates this intersection to some extent as the authors bring their personal perspectives and experiences to bear on the wider research agenda. In Chapter 3, Maureen Lahiff explicitly draws on history to understand the present.

Our other commitment is to examine the relationship between research and practice in an interactive way so as to reveal the importance of practice to inform research and the importance of practice as a form of research. Given the emphasis on evidence-based practice in the current health service research and development strategy we want to look more closely at what counts as 'evidence'. Our examination of the interaction between research and practice will help us to do this by demonstrating how practice can be a prime mover for research rather than research, as is traditionally the case, always being seen as the prime mover for practice.

In the world of market competition and contracts the frontline practitioner may often feel between a rock and a hard place, squeezed between cost efficiency and care. This book's contributors demonstrate the potential of research to enhance knowledge and understanding and negotiate a route to new perspectives and prospects.

The production process

The book came about because Moya Jolley, an experienced colleague, author and editor of nursing texts, approached Pam Smith with the idea for a new look at nursing research. She identified Pam as a potential editor because of her experience of teaching, supervising and undertaking research about nurses, practice and education. With her help, the book proposal began to take shape around the issue of setting agendas and for whom? In seeking contributors for such a book, Pam approached people because of who they were, with particular biographies, expertise and research interests. It is not a coincidence that she had worked with all 11 authors, eight of whom shared the same experience of a health authority committed to promoting a nursing research culture. Those eight authors had not only participated in the positive experience of that culture but had also helped to shape it. The three remaining colleagues and Pam taught and undertook research together in an institution of higher education where we grappled with balancing high teaching loads with scholarly activity. The shared experiences of all the authors underpin these chapters and may be said to shape our own agendas as set out in this book. Our shared experiences and the book chapters illustrate the coming together of history and biography as recommended by C. Wright Mills.

Before beginning the book all the authors met with the publisher's editor, Fiona Goodgame, and agreed some common goals. Everyone went away to write their draft outlines and return them to Pam Smith for feedback and discussion. The interpretation of the chapters by the editor was passed back to the authors for confirmation. Thus, the process of weaving the book together has been an ongoing process which has continued until the final word was written and punctuated. It is interesting that the Portuguese translation for 'full stop' is 'ponto final' which literally means the 'final point'. This indeed transmits the sense of finality when the production of a book is complete.

Setting the scene: rationale, authors and contents

The underlying rationale for the book, its authors and contents are reflected in the sequence and stance of the chapters. Each chapter provided the authors with an opportunity to explore issues dear to them, and as a vehicle for influencing nursing's research agenda.

Colleen Wedderburn Tate was invited to write the first contributor's chapter. Colleen is a leading Black nurse and midwife. She is also President of CWT Enterprises and Co-Founder of the Community Development Foundation. Her work focuses on raising the visibility of Black people and multiethnic minority peoples within society. It was important that she was able to set the tone for a book which explores new research agendas, given the ethnocentric world of both nursing and research. This is a world which is characterized by values that are predominantly White, male and middle class. In the context of agendas, Colleen is able to put the issue of race, marginalization and the legitimation of lay knowledge firmly in focus.

In Chapter 3, Maureen Lahiff analyses the complexities of medical domination, gender and power relationships in nursing. Maureen's contribution to the book comes from her position as a nursing leader. Her career includes pioneering undergraduate studies for registered nurses, holding the position of chief nurse in a London health authority, and a chair in nursing and midwifery. In retirement, she continues her professional career as an independent consultant. Maureen gives an historical context to the setting of agendas and identifies the major influences on and from nursing, education and research.

The author of Chapter 4, Maria Lorentzon, has acted as a mentor to many nurses and midwives, new to research. She was an important influence in setting research agendas for nursing and midwifery at national and regional level. She has a varied career spanning practice, management, research and evaluation. Most recently she has worked as a research manager in a department of general practice and latterly as an independent consultant. Maria brings a sociological perspective to her chapter as she explores where ideas come from and analyses nursing's position in relation to setting national agendas.

Colleen, Maureen and Maria all identify the centrality of power and the need to get behind the politics, values and assumptions which shape nursing and research agendas. In Chapter 5, Abigail Masterson offers discourse analysis as one example of a liberating research method which can assist nurses and others to analyse and shape agendas. Abigail is a committed practitioner in the care of older people. Her academic background is in social policy which she uses to inform her nursing practice, education and research.

The chapters which follow focus on specific issues pertinent to setting research agendas. Gosia Brykczyńska has become something of an expert nurse ethicist, writer and teacher. Her contribution to the book is to raise questions about the morality and ethics of the research process, including the compatibility between nurse as carer and nurse as researcher; the integrity of the findings and their application to practice.

The authors of Chapter 7 in their compelling title 'Researching hidden worlds' continue to explore moral and ethical issues in research as they apply in the field. Trudi James and Dawn Whittaker discuss the interface between the role of practitioner and researcher in the study of sensitive subjects which also touch on their personal and work interests in potentially marginalized groups. Trudi and Dawn were invited to contribute to the book because of their commitment to practitioner and user-led research which they demonstrate in their roles as nurses working with women.

Chapters 8 and 9 are practitioner rather than research-led chapters. The contributors are practitioners who bring research-mindedness to the study of their practice. Helen Mann, an expert ward sister of 20 years standing, uses research to recognize her skills and transfer them to a clinical nurse-specialist role. Anne Jones and Olwyn Bamford, pioneers of what Salvage (1990) refers to as the 'new nursing', describe their involvement in a Nursing Development Unit which could be interpreted as a response to but also a means of setting research agendas. In both chapters the authors explore the meaning of practitioner-led knowledge as opposed to formalized scientific knowledge. They demonstrate the use of research to analyse their practice but also to show how practice can be seen as a form of research, particularly in relation to the generation of knowledge. The chapters also show the intersection of biography and history since the authors write of external changes which impacted both positively and negatively on their personal and professional lives.

These particular chapters were costly in terms of the emotions they evoked for the authors. They also illustrate the difficulties experienced by the other authors, especially those who were primarily practitioners, in finding time and space to reflect and document their experiences. This lack of 'think time' in the labour process is well-documented by authors such as Hales (1980) and is associated with the 'new Taylorism' by which the labour process is fragmented (Braverman, 1974). Consequently, the learning required to do a job, together with the autonomy and discretion required, are discounted.

Chapters 7, 8 and 9 highlight the complexity of nursing work, its interface with research and the invisible aspects of the job associated not only with 'think time' but also emotional labour in negotiating relationships between colleagues, patients and nurses (Smith, 1992).

A number of consistent and discrete themes arise throughout all the chapters. Gender is one such theme. This should not come as too much of a surprise given (a) all the authors are women; (b) nursing is predominantly a woman's occupation. Feminist scholarship has been sharply critical of the systematic bias in academic disciplines which have been dominated by the particular and limited interests, perspectives and experiences of White males (Nielsen, 1990, p. 96).

The themes from all the chapters are drawn together in an epilogue contained in Chapter 10. Pam invited her colleague and friend, Angie Cotter, to co-write this chapter. We had stood in the first United Kingdom Central Council for Nursing, Midwifery and Health Visiting (UKCC) election on a radical nurses' ticket. We still share similar political perspectives and our academic interests are complementary but distinct. Angie brings an analytic psychotherapeutic dimension while Pam's perspective is informed by medical sociology. Our collaboration in the book came from a chance conversation in which we realized as nurses and researchers that we shared many past and present realities as well as hopes and dreams for the future.

The chapter explores the possibility of new agendas drawing on the experiences of both the chapter and book authors, the similarities and differences between psychotherapy and research, definitions of knowledge, changes in nurse education and practice, and the impact of the market, informatics and technology on the organization and delivery of health care. We conclude the chapter and book with proposals for a research agenda to take nursing into the twenty-first century. These proposals consider the need to situate the research agenda within the wider national and international context; the incorporation of emotions into the work and research process; a review of the role of patients/clients and lay carers in research; and an assessment of whether nursing should develop its own unique research methodology or incorporate a plurality of perspectives depending on the nature of the question under study.

A note on how the book can be used

We present the book as an exploration of issues for practitioners, managers, educators and researchers. The chapters can be read independently of each other but they also have interrelated themes. Readers can use them as a means of analysing their own work situation and context, set their own agendas and make their proposals for change. The time is at hand for nurses and midwives to contribute to policies and develop strategies to influence future practice, management, education and research, not only for themselves, but also for patients, clients and multidisciplinary colleagues. Our book is designed to assist that process.

References

Braverman H (1974) *Labor and Monopoly Capital: The Degradation of Work in the Twentieth Century*. Monthly Review Press, New York.

Feyerabend P (1978) *Science in a Free Society*. Verso, London.

Hales M (1980) *Living Thinkwork*. Free Association Books, London.

Kratz C (1978) *Care of the Long-term Sick in the Community: Particularly Patients with Stroke*. Churchill Livingstone, Edinburgh.

Nielsen J (ed.) (1990) *Feminist Research Methods: Exemplary Readings in the Social Sciences*. Westview Press, Boulder, Colorado.

Salvage J (1990) The theory and practice of the 'New Nursing'. *Nursing Times*, Occasional Papers, 86(4), 42–5.

Smith P (1992) *The Emotional Labour of Nursing: How Nurses Care*. Macmillan, Basingstoke.

Wilson-Barnett J (ed.) (1983) Nursing research: ten studies in patient care. *Developments in Nursing Research*, 2. John Wiley, Chichester.

Wright Mills C (1970) *The Sociological Imagination*. Penguin, Harmondsworth.

2

'B' road or motorway? : charting a future for nursing research

Colleen Wedderburn Tate

This chapter traces the origins of western philosophy on which knowledge, truth and scientific endeavours are based, and challenges the notion that this philosophy alone shapes all such endeavours in other societies. The author shows how historians use a variety of sources to arrive at different and often conflicting interpretations of the same event. The 'Black Athena' debate is used to illustrate this point and to ask how is knowledge constructed and on whose terms? What becomes 'fact', what 'fiction' and how do particular concepts survive the passage of time and random nature of history? What is the nature of evidence?

Story telling and oral histories are presented as powerful methods of accessing the hidden history of groups marginalized by gender, race, class or occupation. The author illustrates how, by using story-telling, nurses can challenge the assumptions behind what currently constitutes 'truth' and develop new ways of discovering what drives nursing philosophy and ultimately its evidence-based practice.

Introduction

In the beginning – The Knowledge

In a scene from the television adaptation of Alex Haley's book *Roots*, a group of elderly African men are discussing how to solve a problem related to the survival of their village. One television reviewer was highly critical of this scene, arguing that it was unrealistic and portrayed these men as philosophers, whereas in the context of the time they were probably uneducated and illiterate. Although this review was written nearly two decades ago, the feeling of bewilderment is fresh. What were the assumptions on which the reviewer based the description 'not philosophers'? What pre-knowledge existed to define someone as uneducated or illiterate? And what emotional contact did readers of the review have with the words 'African', 'philosophers', 'uneducated', and 'illiterate'? The scene under review represents actual life in many villages in Africa, and community life elsewhere. Ordinary people frequently discuss issues of great import to their lives without ever having heard of such Western philosophers as Hume, Locke, Descartes or Erasmus.

Similarly, nurses like 'ordinary people' also discuss important issues without having been exposed to courses in philosophy. The introduction of academic topics during educational programmes, particularly at pre-registration level, is still comparatively recent. Like the elders from the African village depicted in the scene above, nurses' voices have not always been valued or listened to by those in power. Yet within their own groups, nurses find no difficulties in finding a language to describe the emotional, intuitive and creative dimensions of their work (Hart, 1991).

The idea that nursing has an oral tradition has a long history. This tradition lends itself to the use of critical incidents and reflection in learning about and developing nursing practice (Clamp, 1980; Schon, 1987). These approaches have become increasingly popular over the past decade, giving nurses both the skills and opportunities to undertake research-based patient care. But like a car-driver who set off to find the M25 and ends up on the B4112, nurses who champion research-based patient care must be wondering why such a relatively simple idea is in danger of being detoured. Furthermore, as nurse education moves into mainstream higher education, the emphasis on acquiring research-based knowledge as a legitimate function will increase.

Nursing's drive for academic credibility and intellectual respectabilty presents the real possibility of widening the gap in the relationship with our patients, and neglecting alternative methods of enquiry which could enhance patients' experience of health care. Many bedside nurses are alarmed by what they see as the rush to secure academic credentials, with no visible impact on standards of patient care. This is a view which has also been expressed by health care managers over time, in the context of 'over-training' nurses (Reverby, 1994).

Nurses remain a marginalized occupational group, primarily because most nurses are women. As Abigail Masterson discusses in Chapter 5, nurses are not a homogenous group but are composed of practitioners, educators, researchers and managers. They are further subdivided by specialty and place of work, but collectively constitute the largest producer group in the health service (Buchan, 1991). This fact therefore should make them a powerful group in influencing change and setting agendas. However, nurses, particularly those working at the grass roots, are predominantly women. Furthermore, women continue to be marginalized in most societies. Nurses therefore need to consider the wider issues raised by this marginalization of their sex and work, and how they are therefore perceived by policy-makers.

Davies (1995) cites Beardshaw and Robinson (1990) to illustrate this point in the introduction to her book *Gender and the Professional Predicament in*

Nursing. She writes that although: '. . . nurses constitute over half the workforce and their services consume around a quarter of total NHS expenditure . . . nursing has been "marginal to the debates that have shaped health policy since 1948" ' (Beardshaw and Robinson, 1990). Davies therefore devotes 'the major subject matter' of her book to investigate the reasons for this neglect of the nation's nurses: why it is that nursing can remain taken for granted and invisible and the ways in which this invisibility is sustained in policy arenas.

The context in which UK nurses currently work – a market-oriented health care system where providers compete for contracts – presents significant challenges to nurse researchers to justify the value and expense of nurses, and convince sceptical colleagues that research is not about ivory towers and flights of fancy. Nurses, along with other clinicians in the NHS, are required to move towards an evidence-base for practice. As part of the same trend they must also pay rigorous attention to the pursuit of clinical effectiveness, a phrase more often equated with 'evidence-based medicine' (a revealing phrase). Both evidence-based health care and clinical effectiveness are key strands in the Department of Health's drive to ensure that they are incorporated into decision-making about the provision of clinical services. Systematic reviews of existing studies are undertaken to produce evidence of cost, and clinical, effectiveness. Such reviews have led to the discontinuation of procedures such as the insertion of grommets and the dilation and curettage procedure for women under the age of 40 (Dunning, McQuay and Milne, 1994). The drive for evidence-based provision of clinical services presents all kinds of dilemmas for the NHS, not least because doctors, nurses, physiotherapists and others are slow to incorporate research results into clinical practice. Clinical effectiveness is based on the notion of 'proof', which is at the heart of 'scientific method'.

However, delivery of care, as opposed to the provision of care, is an art as well as a science, and nurses need to stop and think clearly about some of the implications of accepting the current context of research in the NHS, with its focus on medical modes of enquiry, which favour technology-dominated and quantitative approaches. If nurses are to fully contribute to debates about health and health care – formulation of policy, efficacy of treatments, the relationships between service users and providers, the organization and leadership of health care – we must take a wider view of the processes by which decisions about health care and its resourcing are made, and transform our own understanding about those processes. Adopting a wider view will demand more questioning of the priorities for funding, a greater understanding of the power and political relationships which are played out in policy-making, and taking a leading role in making health care a subject for informed public debate. The changes needed to ensure that nursing survives as a viable part of the UK health care system depend less on pursuing academic debates about nursing research, and more about redefining nursing and patient care as human endeavours which are as important as the managerial, technical and commercial drives of late twentieth-century health care. Nurses must rethink the whole basis on which health care practice is predicated, and construct alternatives which include patients and their families as key providers of knowledge.

Identity through knowledge

Since the early twentieth century, medical men and hospital administrators have dominated the development of hospital-based health care (Davies, 1990). This domination has been associated with the capture of 'scientific medicine', leaving nurses with no science of their own (Stevens, 1989). Writings on nursing history worldwide record nurses' search for an identity separate from, but complementary to, medicine. The primary focus has been on the art of nursing, with an emphasis on the womanly virtue of caring. This notion of nursing was promulgated by Florence Nightingale and continues to inform the behaviour and attitudes of many nurses around the world. Notwithstanding the difficulties in defining 'caring', nursing as the art of caring is a legitimate goal to pursue.

Caring as a mechanism for humanizing health care systems has been underrated. It was precisely because of the 'caring' label of nursing that young, middle-class women could enter nurse training in the nineteenth and early twentieth centuries. For them, nursing was a way of acquiring a livelihood and a virtuous state (Reverby, 1994). However, for nursing to develop, there had to be a change in the education and social outlook of this group. Such developments, however, revealed the tension between the legitimate drive for a seperate identity from medicine, and a reluctance of many nurses to relinquish the 'virtuous woman' view of nursing (Reverby, 1994). This tension holds true for nurses in many parts of the world and, from personal experience, results in an unwillingness to challenge too far the prevailing gender boundaries in health care practice. Consequently, we are often confused by the 'feast and famine' approach of administrators – in times of nursing shortage, nurses are valued; at other times ignored (Smith and Agard, 1997).

Historically, nursing has been closely identified with medicine and draws both social and organizational power from this relationship. In the nineteenth century, nursing was drawn into hospital-based health care by the efforts of Florence Nightingale. With the founding of the Nightingale School, a boundary was created between woman as nurse and woman in the home (Keyzer, 1988). Between the medical men and the newly tenured nurse lay the patient – passive, barely visible, and grateful.

Carpenter (1978) and Garmarnikow (1978) give well-rehearsed arguments for how the relationships between doctors, matrons, nurses and patients, reproduced the patriarchal family structures of Victorian society. For Carpenter (1978) 'what emerged in the voluntary hospital was the reproduction of the wider Victorian class structure based on preconceived notions of the division of labour between the sexes and between women of different classes'. The matron represented the 'lady of the house' who supported her husband (i.e. the doctor) and supervised the servants (i.e. the nurses). The patients represented the children. The doctors were in sole charge of defining who became patients which for Gamarnikow (1978) was indicative of nursing's subordinate position to medicine.

Nurses have now begun to create clearer definitions of what constitutes nursing, and the role of nursing care in an increasingly technology-driven health care system. Initiatives such as the nursing process, primary nursing and nursing development units are evidence of this. The current shift in power within the NHS has put decision-making in the hands of general rather than nurse managers, just as the role of nurses as independent practitioners is being addressed and developed (Keyzer, 1988). This shift threatens to divest nursing of the professional credentials it seeks as illustrated in Chapter 9 by Anne Jones and Olwyn Bamford's account of the rise and fall of a nursing development unit.

A central focus of concern must be the education of nurses. Project 2000 aims to produce the 'knowledgeable doer', an able and educated practitioner able to play a full part in the health care team. One vehicle to develop the 'knowledgeable doer' is a research-base for the practice of nursing. But how do we get to have knowledge of any kind which contributes to this research-base? Where does the knowledge come from? Who, if anyone owns it, guards it, and disposes of it? What impact do the processes of knowledge aquisition have on health care practice, research and development? Questions such as these are beginning to form a substantial part of the debate about the purpose of nurses and nursing, and nurses' contribution to health care. This debate needs to be situated within the context of the development of Western scientific method and a view of knowledge which is the result of that method, based on notions of 'proof' and 'rationality'. This model has come to dominate public and private discourse worldwide, while systematically down-grading other forms of knowledge and knowing, such as story-telling and reflection which would have been familiar to the village elders, depicted at the beginning of this chapter.

Philosophy, knowledge and science

Western philosophy and science have developed as a subjective, individualistic pursuit of knowledge, restricted to a chosen few (Russell, 1962). This model is now breaking down because of a number of factors: increasing rates of literacy worldwide; information technology, which has increased the ability of people to communicate across vast distances; marked disillusionment with what some see as the failure of Western models of science, development, economics and politics; consumerism; feminist and other non-traditional interpretations of history and knowledge.

Russell's *History of Western Philosophy* comprehensively documents the rise of philosophy and science in the West. Although this book was first published 50 years ago, it is still a very useful aid in beginning to understand how Western modes of knowledge and knowing have come to dominate public and private discourse.

Russell argues that philosophy is the bridge between dogma (theology) and science (Russell, 1962). Warburton says that philosophy is 'an activity: ... a way of thinking about certain sorts of questions'(Warburton, 1992). Both these philosophers hold that science is a method of acquiring knowledge: in Russell's case 'definite knowledge'; for Warburton 'truth by authority'. Furthermore, both Russell and Warburton warn of the dangers of a simple view of science as ethically neutral, divorced from the scientist's own world view, and professing to give certainty. However, Western philosophy, theology and science all share a common assumption about the building-blocks that constitute their form: a dominant Western model of what constitutes knowledge and truth.

The branch of philosophy that deals with how knowledge is derived is epistemology. Epistemologists are concerned with theories of the nature of knowledge, how knowledge is tested and validated and whether there are limits to human understanding. The epistemology debate is of particular interest in nursing, as nurses strive to carve out a defining framework of what constitutes nursing knowledge, as opposed to medical knowledge. However, the debate continues to take place in the context of the Western model described above.

The *Black Athena* debate

What is now known as Western civilization had its birth in Greece. However, the foundations of civilization had existed for thousands of years in Mesopotamia (now part of Iraq) and Egypt. Ancient Greek writers documented the impact that colonization by Egyptians and Phoenicians had on the development of their culture. Yet, from the 1820s onwards, Western scholars, notably in Germany and Britain, invented a mode of Greek civilization which ignored what the Greeks themselves had readily acknowleged – that Black and Semitic peoples were instrumental in the development of the religious, economic and cultural life of Greece. The competition between the Western view of Greek civilization (the broad, and extreme, Aryan models), and what the Greeks themselves knew (the Ancient model) has become known as the *Black Athena* debate. This is the title of the exhaustive, and continuing, enquiry by Martin Bernal (1987) into similarities between the Greek vocabulary, and Egyptian and Hebrew. *Black*

Athena charts the influence of Egyptian and Semetic cultures on the formation of Greece in the Middle to Late Bronze Age.

In *Black Athena* Bernal set out, not to 'prove' that the Ancient model is right, but to show that this model is no less plausible than the Aryan model as an explanation of the development of Greek culture and civilization (Bernal, 1987). In volume one (of three) of *Black Athena*, Bernal links the rise of the Aryan model to that of anti-Semitism and the African slave trade. He dates the first systematic efforts to wipe out knowledge of the influence of Egyptians and Jews on Greek culture as 1815–1830. It was also during this period that Christianity was felt to be under threat, Masonic rationalism (early Masons were deeply influenced by Egyptian culture) was suspected in the French Revolution, and many European nations were growing in economic and military power. Clearly, the Ancient model stood in the way of the new belief that Greek culture was, essentially, European, and that civilization and philosophy had orignated in Greece (Bernal, 1987). Prior to this time, it had been widely accepted that Egyptian civilization, which is based on Nubian and Upper Egyptian pre-dynastic cultures (and whose African origins are uncontested) greatly influenced developments in Greek culture and religion. While the ancient Greeks feared and despised Egyptians and Phoenicians, at the same time they had a deep respect for the philosophy and religion of these two cultures.

The concepts of 'progress' (or 'later is better'), professionalism and racialism (what Bernal calls 'the three cardinal beliefs of the nineteenth century') remain today as a bulwark against ideas that threaten deeply held beliefs about the origins of Western civilization. Or to put it another way: 'After the rise of black slavery and racialism, European thinkers were concerned to keep black Africans as far as possible from European civilization' (Bernal, 1987).

The *Black Athena* debate challenges not only nineteenth century received wisdom about European civilization. It also shows how language and, through it, the acquisition of knowledge and knowing, shapes and defines a society. The European thinkers who denied the influence of non-European peoples on Greek culture were also teachers. Their students would have continued in the same vein (given that by the time any subject begins to be understood, the main ideas have usually been passively ingested, without much challenge). *The status quo* is maintained by successive generations of students up to the present day, as they continue to be taught using similar language. Thus is 'knowledge' acquired and perpetuated.

Write it down

The *Black Athena* debate does not obscure the key skill that the Greeks contributed to the development of civilization: writing. The Greeks *wrote down* what they saw, thought and did. Previously, recording of events had been by recital, or annals. Hence, the arrival of documentation had a profound effect on how knowledge was acquired, and who could acquire it. Documentation also served to isolate the public world of men from the private world of women and the home. Whereas a recital of a group's history will contain a sense of how the teller related to events, documentation divorces the personal telling from the recording. Documentary knowledge therefore enables control of perceptions of what is true through the social organization of knowledge. This form of control is evident in nursing practice: if it is not written down, it is not valid (Campbell, 1988).

Early philosophers differed markedly in their views of the source of knowledge. Plato rejected scientific rationalism (getting facts from experiment) and advocated the establishment of fact through argument. Aristotle argued that what we experience through our senses is our only source of knowledge and, by reasoning, we can discover the distinguishing properties of things. In the sixteenth century, Francis Bacon was concerned about systematically seeking mathematical knowledge. In *The Levathian*, Thomas Hobbes attempted to develop a theory of nature, which in some ways echoed Aristotle.

Intellectual life in the nineteenth and twentieth centuries became much more complex as the orthodoxy of the prevailing philosophy was challenged by philosophers like Karl Marx and Friedrich Nietzsche and science grew from a seventeenth-century novelty to a major player in the acquisition of knowledge.

The first half of the twentieth century saw the emergence in Western Europe of demagogic politicians and fascist ideologues such as Hitler and Mussolini. Hitler, for example, used the Aryan model to promote his idea of the 'Master' race which justified the elimination of whole sectors of society including Jews, gypsies, homosexuals, the chronically sick and people with learning disabilities. Thus science and medicine began to be systematically used to denigrate and destroy people or ideas that ran counter to Hitler's Nazi party policies.

Shevell and Evans (1994) note that the conceptual framework of 'racial hygiene' which underpinned Nazism, legitimized the conduct of 'marginal investigations' on individuals who were regarded as defective and genetically inferior. This framework also sanctioned euthanasia and extermination for those considered socially and physically unfit. Psychiatrists were identified by Michael Burleigh (1995) as playing a 'pioneering role ... in the evolution of the Nazis' murderous racial policy' fuelled by anti-Semitism and eugenics.

The Nuremberg trials (December 1946 – August 1947) of 20 physicians and their associates, focused on the atrocities of human experimentation in the concentration camps. The trials showed that: 'Within the context of a state and society that systematically devalued the intrinsic worth of certain classes of human beings, unethical experiments did occur within the ivory tower of academic medicine'.

Although the examples from Hitler's Third Reich may be viewed as extreme, the potential for the scientific method to be used in this way has worrying implications for the development of a humane research approach which recognizes the diversity of the human race.

Science in the late twentieth century has come full circle, with scientists exploring the nature of God, the universe and everything. While schools strive to make science interesting and fun, radio programmes such as *Science Now* place science as a long-standing part of everyday life and books like a *A Brief History of Time* become best-sellers. The modern scientist is the new hero, as witnessed by the acclaim for physicist Andrew Wiles for solving Fermat's Last Theorem.

In a Radio 4 programme, Steven Rose, Professor of Biology at the Open University, and presenter of the 1995 BBC/Open University lecture, was invited to discuss with other studio guests the public images of science and how they were handled by television and the visual media. Rose was critical of the gendered and élitist view of science which predominated. His criticisms included some of the following comments:

> In both TV fiction and the factual treatment of science, what turns up again and again is the incredibly male authoritative voice. Women on the whole, are not shown as TV presenters of science, except for kids, but rather as helpless, squeaky 'side kicks' to the scientist of power embodied in such sci-fi characters as 'Dr Who' and 'Quatermass'.

Rose's concern was whether this was a 'true' vision of science. He concluded that women were excluded from TV and the visual media so that it appeared overwhelmingly that the majority of science was done, and spoken for, by men.

Rose continued:

> I think it happens because there are processes within science which achieve this exclusion and are reinforced by television images. The other thing that happens is that you are never allowed to learn within the context of television about the social processes of science. You are never allowed to believe that there is doubt, there is controversy. There is this emphasis on certainty which comes through. TV does considerable harm both to science and the media and if you get a more open science, a science which interacts with non-scientists, then you need to get a better two-way dialogue between the scientists and the rest of society and that is what television is failing to do.
>
> The point about scientists and what they do is that they generate power and authority. They claim to tell us how the world is and how we are supposed to think, and in so far that television simply reflects that and produces these all powerful images, it does an important disservice. What the media says and does is enormously influential.

Studio guest (Tariq Ali) cited one important exception to the trend:

> There has been one very exciting TV drama about the struggle for DNA which did popularize that particular struggle in which a woman scientist's (Rosalind Franklin) role was acknowledged and how she'd been done out of it (the Nobel

prize) by the boys at Cambridge (Crick and Watson). But in general Steven is right.

(For background to this struggle read Sayre A (1975) *Rosalind Franklin and DNA.* Norton, New York).

Rose's critique does not hide the fact that, by and large, the language of science remains incomprehensible to, and excludes, most people. So while science may have come of age, the scientific method of enquiry is still male-dominated and informs the way knowledge is sought, acquired and accessed. Similarly, in medicine, the mechanistic view of the human body is emphasized; women are pathologized and the private world of ill health is turned into a public discourse founded on hospital-based health care dominated by medical men.

Nursing, nurses, and research

As far back as 1972, the Briggs Report advocated that nursing become a research-based profession. Since that time, there have been many other reports advocating the same development. The NHS reforms of 1991 have accelerated such calls. The need for a research-base in nursing is, variously, to achieve accountability (Bircumshaw, 1990), to establish evidence-based practice (DoH, 1993), and to integrate nursing research into clinical activity (Shuldham, 1996). Another key factor in the development of a clear structure and agenda for nursing research is to secure funding. In Chapter 4 in this book, Maria Lorentzon argues that the degree to which nurses, and other health care professionals, can determine their own research agendas, and attract funding, will be a reflection of their overall influence within the NHS, and in society in general.

How far have nurses managed to get their agenda for research into the sights of decison-makers, and have nurses done enough to ensure that they have a voice in health care policy?

Power and presence

As Lorentzon points out, nurses hold very few places on research and development (R&D) committees, and none as chair. A similar condition would seem to prevail in the USA. The Agency for Health Care Policy and Research, an organization established to develop clinical guidelines, appears to have only three nurses in chair or co-chair positions, out of a total of seven panels (Warner, 1994). The focus of most R&D committees is firmly on the 'R', and on quantitative methods of finding it. Nursing is caught between the twin goals of developing practice based on some definition of caring, with its qualitative and development overtones, and seeking intellectual credibility by placing nursing education in universities, and creating senior academic posts. Going unaddressed is the inherent conflict between a view of the world which equates legitimacy with published research, which degrades the importance of anecdote and verbal reporting, excludes the reality of women, Blacks, the disabled, the elderly, and the young, and the caring context in which health care delivery presumably operates. It is these neglected groups of people that nurses must bring to the attention of policy-makers and research-funders, and define a workable agenda for different forms of enquiry.

Generally, nurses have an underdeveloped understanding of policy-making. Nurses must be educated to know that public policy-making involves choices with limited resources and between competing objectives. Nurses must accept that conflict, negotiation and compromise are part of the process of influencing policy-making (Larsen, 1988). Therefore, nurses need to be skilled in politics, have the energy to pursue their agendas, and have some form of power (Mintzberg, 1983). However, nurses have as much to lose as to gain from getting close to policy-making. The values, attitudes and language of decision-making is not set by nurses. In the UK this is the province of civil servants. Therefore nurses who want to influence policy must become part of a consensus, and may eventually cease to have a focus on nursing (White, 1988). This is precisely the complaint of many clinical nurses who lament the demise of the 'nurses' nurse'. However, the involvement of nurses in policy-making need not involve a dilution of their role in their professional organizations, or as advocates of their profession. Nurses can influence policy-makers and maintain a focus on nursing by being aware of the values, attitudes and agenda of decision-makers. There is a great difference between simply sitting at the top table, and making a powerful contribution to the processes which drive nursing care. The difference is leadership.

Worries about senior nurses leaving their colleagues behind (Traynor, 1995), the failure of nurse leadership (Nursing Management, 1995), and general concerns about some of the pitfalls of leadership (Dean, 1995), form a significant part of the debate in many nursing journals. However, the leadership required to secure the future of nursing research demands a discourse which is framed by how patients experience health care, and how nurses themselves experience their practice.

Creating a humane research agenda

The placebo effect is the term used to describe the action of a treatment which is not attributable to a pharmological reaction (Watts, 1992). Given that for much of medical history, even today, we know very little about the real effect of any medication, the placebo effect should be just as valid as a result obtained from the physical properties of a drug. This relationship between patient and healer is often dismissed as not valid. However, in

Chapter 10, Cotter and Smith draw on Shapiro's (1995) psychotherapy research to show how the need for a good working relationship between client and therapist requires the placebo effect to be *included* in the research design.

Indeed, in double-blind trials, the elimination of the placebo effect is common practice. Generally, medicine continues to disregard the effect of a person's state of mind on their physical condition. Also disregarded are methods of relating personal histories of health and illness which do not conform to scientific methods of enquiry. For example, when taking medical histories, many doctors and nurses frequently interrupt patients' tales of how they acquired that history. Further, patients' life histories are rarely part of data collection on admission to hospital. Nurses have also failed at this, and no more so than in the early day of the nursing process, with its models of care. Models of care give significant power to nurses to plan, implement and review a patient's care, and further remove the patient as the centre of care (Keyzer, 1988).

Conversely, nurses still feel the need to justify sitting and talking to patients. While the results of these exchanges are often incorporated into the care plan, they are infrequently used as markers for understanding more fully how a patient experienced a particular episode of illness or health. From personal recollection, nurses and midwives are reluctant to cross the line between the patient as recipient of care, and the patient as a person with a unique biography and history: the patient as the story-teller of their life. In Chapter 10, Cotter and Smith suggest that encouraging patients to tell their stories may be seen in the context of 'new' paradigms for caring research.

Telling stories

Story-telling and biography are powerful methods of accessing hidden histories. Contemporary writers and accomplished story-tellers, like Maya Angelou, have proved that the history of a life is made more immediate and moving by listening to the voice of those to whom the related events happened. The work of earlier story-tellers, such as Herodotus' account of the Persian Wars, and Thucydides (the *Black Athena* debate would lead us to observe that his writings exclude mention of Egypt and Phoenicia), can still excite the imagination and vividly bring to life events that occurred thousands of years ago. Such histories are an important part of understanding how people make sense of their circumstances, and how they attempt to control events in their lives.

Oral history can also take the form of allegory. One example is John Bunyan's *Pilgrim's Progress* which describes life as a journey. The *Anancy* stories which are familar to people from all cultures (although different names might be used to describe the main character) is an example of how social mores are passed on through generations. It seems that we are willing to accept oral history as a legitimate form of literature, yet reluctant to apply its obvious contribution to personal definitions of health and illness.

Instead, 'man-made language' is used to lessen the importance of oral history or 'human' language. The presence of 'man-made language' (Spender, 1980) is a powerful oppressor in the lives of women and other groups excluded from the mainstream of decisions and knowledge acquisition. Masterson also notes in Chapter 5 that language can be used as a vehicle for social control and domination. The increasing power of documentary knowledge in nursing leaves little room for nurses to reflect on their lived experiences as workers and providers of care. When nursing is considered in the context of 'women's work', there is a further dilemma as women's issues remain at the margins of health care research.

Despite some changes, nursing continues to be an adjunct to medicine. In a major report on research and development in the NHS (Department of Health, 1994), only passing mention was made to nursing or other non-medical research. As Lorentzon points out in Chapter 4, an interview with the NHS Chief Executive of the day did not include reference to nursing research. These two examples are a reflection of the fact that the organization of and control of health care is formulated on the values of the organizers and controllers (Orr, 1988).

Other writers point to the role that nurses and midwives play in sustaining and maintaining the dominant mode of health care practice and policy (Rich, 1977; Daly, 1979; Oakley, 1980). Yet, by nature of being employed to deliver government policy, nurses are public employees, and therefore work in the realm of politics. At practitioner level, this reality is very evident, especially after the NHS reforms of 1991. Today nurses are not just public employees, but politicized employees operating in an ideology-driven, market-based, efficiency-oriented system of healthcare. By a judicious mix of compromise and appeals to the sanctity of clinical judgement, physicians have always found ways to maintain their agenda in the face of policies presumed to be hostile to their interests.

Conversely, nurses have been relatively easily sidetracked by the apparent gains obtained from Project 2000, higher education, and promises of more active involvement in decision-making. However, it is noticeable that general management demolished the middle level of nurse management, and disputes over clinical regradings have sapped the energies of many nurses. The current furious debate about the rise of bureaucracy in the NHS may be another setback for nurses as non-nurse decision-makers tackle the latest government blitz on management costs by demolishing several layers of clinical nurse managers. Nurses seem destined to be caught looking the other way when decisions about the direction, content and context of health care are made. Nurses must create a clear framework for developing qualitative methods of enquiry into aspects of health care which are not always amenable to experiment or testing, but which provide rich seams of experience.

Learning for care

One of the hidden outcomes of the way knowledge is produced is the continued marginalization of certain groups. The case of women has been discussed above and documented in several publications. More recently, the way Black people, as users and employees, experience society and social systems, including the health care system, has become a subject of debate both in the UK and the USA (Floyd, 1992; Walker, 1992; Nzegwu, 1993). Such studies, frequently conducted by Black researchers with a strong focus on participation isssues, are only just being 'legitimized' by publication in mainstream journals, and by major publishers. In the USA the discourse on the *Black Athena* debate is confined to a limited group of academics and researchers.

More in the public arena is a long-standing debate about the existence of a Black philosophy of history, medicine and nursing. As would be expected, the lines of argument are much more developed in the USA, with its larger population of Black people. The focus of debates in the US is the process by which Black history, knowledge and intellectual activity was subordinated by the belief in the inferior nature of Black people as a race.

Because documentation, and belief in the written word, plays such a strong part in scientific method, some early explorers to Africa felt free to offer written interpretations of what they saw, having little understanding of how their previously constructed frameworks about what was true affected their perceptions. Hence, rituals or practices which were not obviously European were dismissed as 'mumbo-jumbo', or the consequence of loose morals. Because any system is underpinned by the values and attitudes of those who organize it, it is not difficult to understand why colonization and slavery happened, why ancient civilizations were ransacked for profit, and why native peoples in Australia, the USA and Canada are still explaining why it is not appropriate to build office blocks, or other commercial enterprises, on their tribal burial grounds.

The use of history as a distorting mirror is amply illustrated by the history of racialism in Western thought. There are people who continue to hold to the belief that the Holocaust was a myth, that Africans did not mind being enslaved, that race determines intelligence, and that men are the natural leaders under any circumstances. Given that such beliefs form part of a given social morality, it stands that some nurses may also hold such views. If this is true (in the sense of being able to be proved), then enquiry into the health care needs of denigrated groups will not form part of some nurses' agenda. Even in the realm of everyday care, the stories that such patients may tell may be ignored. This is illustrated by two cases from personal experience.

During a history-taking session on a gynaecological ward, a doctor was heard by all the other women verbally and racially abusing a Black woman patient, who was partially deaf. This conversation was also heard by two staff nurses standing at the nurses' desk. When challenged to support the woman, the nurses claimed that the woman was 'difficult to communicate with' and the particular doctor was 'always like that'. One of the nurses stated that she had not heard anything. This case falls within continued attempts by many nurses to maintain a *status quo* where their daily working relationships become more important than the well-being of patients. There is no suggestion that this is done deliberately. However, given the failure of the NHS over many years to be sensitive and responsive to patients' needs, it should be no surprise that, in circumstances such as those described above, many nurses take the line of least resistance. What could also have been operating was the staff nurses' sub-conscious agreement with the physician's attitudes about people who were Black and/or deaf.

In the second case, a consultant obstetrician failed to attend a non-English speaking, non-White woman, who was having a difficult labour. Despite repeated requests from the midwives, the obstetrician refused to intervene (because she wasn't 'his' patient). The baby was stillborn, and no action was taken against either the consultant or the midwives (but the incident is still talked about). Again, the reluctance of 'mere midwives' to challenge the behaviour of a consultant has many of its roots in the continued subservience of nursing to medicine; and, probably, in the fact that the woman was non-White.

Both these cases illustrate the ethical dilemmas which nurses meet as a matter of routine in their daily practice. Documentary procedures do not always provide a satisfactory route for nurses to address such lived experiences. Or rather, nurses do not always recognize that the unethical behaviour, or act of racialism, can be recorded in the official documentation. Research in health care is so constructed that the telling of such 'stories' by nurses, women and others, is passed over as anecdote and of little consequence or merit. And anyway, where is the *actual* proof that the incident happened? Nurses themselves aid and abet this negation of personal history and knowledge by looking for knowledge and truth in journals and textbooks. The belief that research-based nursing requires considerable post-qualification study (Chapman, 1996) needs to be qualified. Academic study must lead to a humane understanding of patients' experience of care. It need not take place in the traditional setting of a university classroom or lecture hall, and should not presume that scientific method is the only process of acquiring this knowledge.

Nurses may wish to design clinical practices which put people at the heart of health care. In a real sense, health service users are as marginalized as nurses. The difference is that nurses can make a grab for power through pursuing research-based knowledge. All the rest have to offer is a messy reality which may make the listener uncomfortable, angry and defensive. Black patients do not expect to be treated with respect when they use health services (for example, issues about personal care, religious needs, and skin and hair care are still not given the attention they deserve) because the reality of their social experiences is a lack of respect for their culture and colour. Women, who are the main users of health services, are often patronized or ignored by medical staff, and sometimes by nurses and midwives.

In a study of the effects of social support on mothers of low-birth-weight babies, Ann Oakley (1989), a feminist sociologist, demonstrated that these attitudes and behaviours biased the selection of research subjects. In Oakley's experience, the use of randomized controlled trials and random numbers have advantages over human intuition in reducing bias. She states:

> Human beings are not always right in the judgements they make. The pro-
> fessional ideology of midwifery along with that of other health professionals,
> has been shown to lead to discriminatory stereotyping of women, based on
> such characteristics as working class or ethnic minority. (Macintyre, 1976;
> Graham and Oakley, 1981)

The reality of women's experience, therefore, especially if they are Black, is that they are treated as inferior to men. Disabled people may not even be able to physically access health care premises. Many elderly people have a social experience of being discarded because of their age. The views and experiences of children and young people are generally ignored, except in the context of being the victims of health care rationing, or drug-dealers. The social experience of marginalization is also by class, by language, by dress, by location and by medical condition. Take all this away, and what is left are the clean, tangible, high-status medical conditions whose treatment and diagnosis are amenable to the positivist, linear model of enquiry or mode 1 knowledge (described by Cotter and Smith in Chapter 10).

The notion of 'clean, tangible, high-status medical conditions' is illustrated by Kelly and May's (1982) extensive critique of the literature on 'good' and 'bad' patients. They found that patients with certain illnesses, diseases and symptoms were more or less popular with doctors and nurses. The patients' popularity also depended on their age, gender, race and class characteristics. The most popular patients were those who were young and suffering from curable conditions.

Biography and lived experience are not easily amenable to the restrictive definitions of mode 1 knowledge associated with traditional scientific method. Both are part of everyday life, which is the laboratory of the qualitative researcher (Morse, 1994). Qualitative research relies on insight, luck, logic and inference, which eventually leads to some coherent end-result. Indeed, medicine developed informally over many centuries of carefully recording the patterns of people's illnesses (Morse, 1994). Several biographies and autobigraphies detail the role that 'magic' and intuition played in scientific breakthroughs (Watson, 1980; Crick 1988; Hawking, 1988). Cotter and Smith cite Wertheim's observation that historically, science and magic are closely associated. Indeed, alchemy – the pursuit of turning base metals into gold – was the forerunner of modern day metallurgy. Magic, as an intuitive method in qualitative research, has parallels with work on how nurses exercise expert clinical judgement (May, 1994). It is also about being able to move freely between the concrete and the abstract: to expose the learning in books to the 'real world' where data are produced. Nurses need to find a way to incorporate biography and story-telling into a strong, creative framework for conducting health care research. They also need to find ways to reduce the harm which has been caused by the insensitive application of scientific method.

One possible way to do this is to rediscover a passion for caring. This will become more important as developments in health care provison and delivery become more remote, literally, from patients. For example, tele-medicine has the potential to treat large numbers of patients without physical contact with a health care worker. In some specialities, physicians are now able to consult about patient care with colleagues in another part of the country (or even the world) by interactive television, while the patient is being treated. While such developments will certainly make use of scarce health care resources, it makes nurses and physicians increasingly semi-detached from their patients. In the wider society, the Internet/information super-highway, and virtual reality, presents a danger that we may all become so physically divorced from each other, that opportunities for the sharing and consolidation of experiences will decrease.

A passion for patient care demands that we are present with our patients: that is, we are able to understand what makes them tick. Interestingly, one of the unresolved issues arising from using nursing models, and from different ways of organizing the delivery of nursing care, is the obvious stress that nurses and midwives experience by concentrated contact with patients. The task-allocation approach had the advantage that once the task was done, a nurse could legitimately disappear into the sluice or treatment room. While nursing models and primary midwifery/nursing have probably improved the psychological care of patients, they have also sapped the emotional energies of many midwives and nurses. Therefore, there needs to be a balance between the twin legitimacies of increasing passion in patient care delivery, and protecting health care workers from some of the side-effects of this intense involvement. To date, health care systems have abandoned passion in favour of the 'objective' pursuit of research-based knowledge.

The limits of research

Lee (1993) cites Bell and Encell who argue that 'sociology is done *on* the relatively powerless *for* the relatively powerful'. The organization of social research limits enquiry into powerful groups in society. However, if proposals which are deemed sensitive are not presented, not reviewed, not considered, and therefore not funded, then limits to enquiry become a self-fulfilling prophecy (Lee, 1993). This does not change the fact that research as currently organized in most disciplines takes a linear, positivistic and quantitative approach. This approach is aided by the narrow, short-term agenda of policy-making. Even when attempts are made to involve patients in decisions about their care, the results are not necessarily to patients' benefit. Allshouse (1993) argues that clinical decision models, which aim to help patients decide the relative utility of each outcome in a decision tree, are not fool-proof. Patients may not know how to place a 'value' on outcomes like disability or pain if they have no prior experience of these. Furthermore, how a question is put, the mood of the patient at the time of the decision, and the patient's emotional response to certain questions may affect the decision. While clinical decision models help to clarify alternatives, and identify areas of uncertainty, they may also contain system or human errors which are overly optimistic about some outcomes.

Qualitative research is also not without its limitations. Clarke (1992, 1995), for example, criticizes selected nursing research studies for their lack of rigour and generalizability. Qualitative researchers are becoming increasingly conscious that if their preferred approaches are to be acceptable to the research community in general, a number of appropriate evaluative standards which address issues of systematic rigour need to be devised on which they can be judged (Morse and Field, 1996).

Nurses need to think more deeply and clearly about the import of research in patients' lives, and involve them more closely in the planning and delivery of research. It is not acceptable for nurses to pursue a research agenda which has as one focus to play 'catch-up' with physicians who, because their research tradition is at least four centuries old, are seen as superior in some way. The question is, 'How much of research by physicians is used, and usable?'. The Office of Technology Assessment (1978) estimated that only 15% of medical practice is based on research. Technology assessment is now part of the wider NHS research agenda for the development of evidence-based medicine. While nursing research may have a much shorter history than that of medical research, we need to review what impact that research has had over that time, and be aware that nursing research will increasingly be subjected to the same 'proof' standards as medicine. Therefore, the debate about nursing research should be about the role of nurses in enabling patients' lived care experiences to be expressed in health care policy, and how this enables its effective provision and delivery. The research method adopted will reflect the outcomes of these conversations. One of the dangers of the current focus on clinical effectiveness through evidence-based practice is that the NHS appears to assume that the work of health care organizations alone can improve physical and mental health. Magic, in the form of creativity and insight, can only be a reality in health care research if there is colloboration between all the agencies that impact on people's lives. This does not mean a wholesale move to multidisciplinary research programmes, but more a considered and thoughtful view of how the actions of public and private agencies are implicated in creating many of the problems research sets out to solve.

Nurses face significant challenges in defining and understanding their role in a post-industrial, information-overloaded society. Our roles as individuals, practitioners and citizens intersect and cannot be viewed in isolation from each other. Therefore, nurses must find ways to bring the experience of all three roles to discussions about health care policy and research. We must be leaders in society as well as in clinical practice. We must work to decrease the growing gap between ourselves and our patients. We must also work to repair the damage done to our working relationships with each other by the random pursuit of intellectual credibility and respectability. To seek ways to improve our practice, to desire intellectual growth, to advocate rigorous analysis of what we do and how we do it, are all legitimate activities. We must not achieve these goals at the expense of the humanity of patients, our colleagues and ourselves.

References

Allshouse K D (1993) Treating patients as individuals. In Gerteis M, Edgman-Levitan S, Daley J, Delbanco T L (eds) *Through the Patient's Eyes: Understanding and Promoting Patient-centred Care*. Jossey Bass, San Francisco: 19–44.

Beardshaw V and Robinson K (1990) *New for Old? Prospects for Nursing in the 1990s*, Research Report 8. King's Fund Institute, London.

Bernal M (1987) *Black Athena: The Afroasiatic Roots of Classical Civilization* (Volume 1). Rutgers University Press, New Jersey.

Bircumshaw D (1990) The utilisation of research findings in clinical nursing practice. *Journal of Advanced Nursing* 15: 1272–80.

Buchan J (1991) Assessing the cost of nursing. *Nursing Standard* 6(4): 40.

Burleigh M (1995) *Death and Deliverance: 'Euthanasia' in Germany 1900–1945*. Cambridge University Press, Cambridge.

Campbell M L (1988) Accounting for care: analysing change in Canadian nursing. In White R (ed.) *Political Issues in Nursing: Past, Present and Future* (Volume 3). John Wiley, Chichester: 45–70.

Carpenter M (1978) Mangerialism and the division of labour in nursing. In Dingwall R and McKintosh J (eds) *Readings in the Sociology of Nursing*. Churchill Livingstone, Edinburgh.

Chapman H (1996) Why do nurses not make use of a solid research base? *Nursing Times* 17(92): 38–9.

Clamp C (1980) Learning through incidents. *Nursing Times* 76(40): 1755–8.

Clarke L (1992) Qualitative research: meaning and language. *Journal of Advanced Nursing* 17: 243–52.

Clarke L (1995) Nursing research: science, visions and telling stories. *Journal of Advanced Nursing* 21: 584–93.

Crick F (1988) *What Mad Pursuit: A Personal View of Scientific Discovery.* Basic Books, New York.

Daly M (1979) *Gynaecology.* The Women's Press, London.

Davies C (1995) *Gender and the Professional Predicament in Nursing.* Open University Press, Buckingham.

Davies K (1990) *Women and Time: Weaving the Strands of Everyday Life.* Avebury, Aldershot.

Dean D (1995) Leadership: The Hidden Dangers. *Nursing Standard* 10:12–14, 54–5.

Department of Health (1993) *Targeting Practice: The Contribution of Nurses, Midwives and Health Visitors to the Health of the Nation.* HMSO, London.

Department of Health (1994) *Supporting Research and Development in the NHS (Culyer Report).* HMSO, London.

Dunning M, McQuay H and Milne R (1994) Getting a GRIP. *Health Services Journal* 104(5400) April 28: 24–5.

Floyd V D (1992) 'Too soon, too small, too sick': black infant mortality. In Braithwaite R L and Taylor S E (eds) *Health Issues in the Black Community.* Josey-Bass, San Francisco: 165–77.

Gamarnikow E (1978) Sexual division of labour: the case of nursing. In Kuhn A and Wolpe A M (eds) *Feminism and Materialism: Women and Modes of Production,* Routledge & Kegan Paul, London.

Graham H and Oakley A (1981) Competing ideologies of reproduction: medical and maternal perspectives on pregnancy and birth. In Roberts H (ed) *Women, Health and Reproduction.* Routledge & Kegan Paul, London.

Hart L (1991) Ghost in the machine. *Health Services Journal* 101: 20–2.

Hawking S W (1988) *A Brief History of Time: From Big Bang to Black Holes.* Guild Publishing, London.

Kelly M P and May D (1982) Good and bad patients: a review of the literature and a theoretical critique. *Journal of Advanced Nursing* 7(2): 147–57.

Keyzer D M (1988) Challenging role boundaries: conceptual frameworks for understanding the conflict arising from the implementation of the nursing process in practice. In White R (ed.) *Political Issues in Nursing: Past, Present and Future* (Volume 3). John Wiley, Chichester: 95–119.

Larsen J L (1988) Being powerful: from talk to action. In White R (ed.) *Political Issues in Nursing: Past, Present and Future* (Volume 3). John Wiley, Chichester: 1–13.

Lee R M (1993) *Doing Research on Sensitive Topics.* Sage, London.

Macintyre S (1976) To have or have not: promotion and prevention in gynaecological work. In Stacey M (ed.) *The Sociology of the NHS.* Sociological review monograph 22, University of Keele, Staffordshire.

May K A (1994) Abstract knowing: the case for magic in method. In Morse J M (ed.) *Critical Issues in Qualitative Research.* Sage, London: 10–21.

Mintzberg H (1983) *Power In and Around Organizations.* Prentice-Hall, New Jersey.

Morse J M (1994) Qualitative research: fact or fantasy? In Morse J M (ed.) *Critical Issues in Qualitative Research.* Sage, London: 1–7.

Morse J M and Field P A (1996) *Nursing Research: The Application of Qualitative Research Approaches*, 2nd edn. Chapman & Hall, London.

News (1995) Profession 'losing self-control', *Nursing Management*, 2:7, 4.

Nzegwu F (1993) *Black People and Health Care in Contemporary Britain*. International Institute for Black Research, Reading.

Oakley A (1980) *Women Confined*. Martin Robertson, London.

Oakley A (1989) Who's afraid of the randomized controlled trial? Some dilemmas of the scientific method and 'good' research practice. *Women and Health* 15(4): 25–57.

Orr J (1988) Women's health: a nursing perspective. In White R (ed.) *Political Issues in Nursing: Past, Present and Future* (Volume 3). John Wiley, Chichester: 121–37.

Reverby S (1994) A caring dilemma: womanhood and nursing in historical perspective. In Hein E C and Nicholson M J (eds) *Contemporary Leadership Behaviour*. J B Lippincott, Philadelphia: 3–15.

Rich A (1977) *Of Woman Born*. Virago, London.

Russell B (1962) *History of Western Philosophy*. Allen & Unwin, London.

Schon D A (1987) *Educating the Reflective Practitioner*. Jossey Bass, San Francisco.

Shapiro D (1995) Finding out how psychotherapies help people change. *Psychotherapy Research* 5(1): 1–21.

Shevell M I and Evans B K (1994) The 'Schaltenbrand experiment', Wurzburg, 1940: Scientific, historical and ethical perspectives. *Neurology* 44: 350–6.

Shuldham C (1996) Introducing an integrated nursing research programme. *Nursing Standard* 10:18, 42–3.

Smith P and Agard E (1997) Care costs: towards a critical understanding of care. In Brykczyńska G (ed.) *Caring – The Compassion and Wisdom of Nursing*. Arnold, London.

Spender D (1980) *Man-made Language*. Routledge & Kegan Paul, London.

Stevens R (1989) *In Sickness and in Wealth: American Hospitals in the Twentieth Century*. Basic Books, New York.

Traynor M (1995) Nurse executives: buying in or selling out? *Nursing Management* 2:6, 8–10.

Walker B (1992) Health policies and the black community. In Braithwaite R L and Taylor S E (eds) *Health Issues in the Black Community*. Josey-Bass, San Francisco: 315–20.

Warburton N (1992) *Philosophy: The Basics*. Routledge, London.

Warner D C (1994) Nursing and public policy: what is the high ground? In Hein E C and Nicholson M J (eds) *Contemporary Leadership Behaviour*. J B Lippincott, Philadelphia: 453–60.

Watson J (1980) *The Double Helix: A Personel Account of the Discovery of the Structure of DNA*. Norton, New York.

Watts G (1992) *Pleasing the Patient*. Faber & Faber, London.

White R (1988) The influence of nursing on the politics of health. In White R (ed.) *Political Issues in Nursing: Past, Present and Future* (Volume 3). John Wiley, Chichester: 15–31.

Further reading

Bernal M (1987) *Black Athena: The Afroasiatic Roots of Classical Civilization* (Volume 2). Rutgers University Press, New Jersey.

Gaarder J (1995) *Sophie's World*. Phoenix House, London.
Hogwood B W and Gunn L A (1984) *Policy Analysis for the Real World*. Oxford University Press, Oxford.
Seedhouse D (1991) *Liberating Medicine*. John Wiley, Chichester.
Street A (1995) *Nursing Replay: Researching Nursing Culture Together*. Churchill Livingstone, London.

3

Nursing research: 'The why and the why not'?

Maureen Lahiff

The aim of this chapter is to introduce the reader to some issues in the development of nursing research in the United Kingdom. It draws on the author's personal studies and experiences during the decades which have seen nursing research blossom.

Using the published material of some of the professions' pioneer researchers a picture emerges of their struggles and successes; of the role of the profession and the culture in which nursing operates. The constant question for the reader to bear in mind is 'Who was setting the research agenda here?', 'Who supported or opposed this individual, this policy, this idea?'

By questioning what underlies the descriptions we have of any historical event we may achieve insights into why things are as they are, and why obstacles appear in unexpected times and places. Studying pioneer work is also inspirational; we can take heart from the achievements of others which enables us to press on and overcome the obstructions we face today.

Introduction

Like medicine, with which it has a symbiotic relationship, nursing has a long history. It has developed haphazardly with knowledge passed down within families and communities until the last century, when the roots of professions as we know them today were laid down. To some extent they still suffer from the cultural constraints of that time. Victorian society was dominated by the worship of progress by state, civil, military and church institutions controlled and maintained by men. Engineering, science, medicine are only a few of the occupations which continue to be male-dominated; they all grew rapidly as scientific knowledge became available.

The role of women in this process was either that of supporting male endeavours by managing the home, or by working long hours in domestic or factory employment. Upper- and middle-class women worked at home for their keep; lower-class women worked for low wages outside the home. In both cases their work was undervalued by society at large.

The stories of women who broke through into male domains show them to be people of considerable courage. Many readers will be familiar with the story of Florence Nightingale's perseverance in her ambition to become a nurse. The story of Elizabeth Garrett Anderson's fight to become a doctor was even more difficult. Pioneers like her and Sophie Jex-Blake challenged the *status quo*. Manton, Garrett Anderson's biographer, states:

> Women had been excluded successively from the medical guilds, the Royal Colleges and good professional practice, even in midwifery, so that the development of medical education and ethics alike had passed them by. By 1860 the prospects for any woman who wished to win a qualification in medicine in this country were more daunting than ever before. Vested interest, prejudice and custom, so potent in British society, were all against her. (Manton, 1965, p. 66)

Elizabeth, with the support of family and friends, entered the Middlesex Hospital in 1860 prepared to be a nurse for six months as a preliminary to becoming a medical student. She made an ally of the Dean, who was impressed by her intelligent interest in medical work. But students of the time were less than helpful and in conjunction with many medical practitioners, they prevented her formal admission to the medical school. Their reasons included such phrases as:

> the presence of young females as passive spectators in the operating theatre is an outrage on our natural instincts and feelings and calculated to destroy those sentiments of respect and admiration with which the opposite sex is regarded by all right-minded men. (Manton, 1965, p. 352)

It took Elizabeth Garrett Anderson many years to achieve her ambition and she faced many insults; she eventually overcame all the obstacles and completed her studies, though initially she was barred from all official medical posts.

Some of the battles fought by such pioneers have been emulated by nurses who chose to break out of the stereotypical image of the nurse as an obedient, non-thinking, non-reading doctor's assistant. They became thinking, questioning, professional people, able to identify and analyse the components of nursing problems, and conduct rigorous research into establishing a robust knowledge-base for practice, in conjunction with the essential skills needed for clinical practice.

Various topics are introduced to illustrate the development of nursing research. The achievements of pioneers in research and education, experiences of resistance or apathy to new ideas, or solutions to recognized problems. The organization of health care is explored, with its traditional gender division of labour, the dominance of medicine and the subservience of nursing; the tensions which have developed as women in general have laid claim to equal opportunities in all spheres of life.

Drawing on the work of specific writers, the extent to which significant groups among nurse leaders recognized problems within the profession yet, collectively at least, seemed unable to make significant changes in aspects of nursing management and education is noticed. One result of what is described as a paralysing ambivalence left innovation to individuals. Both in research and education, individuals pursued new agendas, creating opportunities for nurses to become graduates and to learn research skills and knowledge. The experiences of nurse researchers in the 1970s is used to give a flavour of more recent times. The highs and lows of a newer generation of pioneers is described, much of it in their own words.

The chapter concludes with a brief discussion of power, autonomy and control, using more recent research findings to provide insights into the ongoing tensions between medicine and nursing as professional boundaries are challenged and changed. Like all the other issues raised there is only a brief and necessarily incomplete array of evidence. Hopefully the ideas presented will encourage readers to explore some of them more deeply. Others may just be glad to be introduced to a broader picture of the context of nursing practice, and therefore to nursing research and how all this relates to setting new agendas.

The threads presented here are used to draw together a woven picture, to make a particular piece of cloth which reflects the many colours affecting the activity of nursing research: agendas, topics, processes, methodologies. All of these and much more make a picture which changes according to the angle from which it is examined.

The past

The development of nursing research in the United Kingdom has been documented by its pioneers, for example Simpson, the first nurse to hold the office of nursing officer (research) at the Department of Health and Social Security (DHSS) in England. In a lecture given in 1971 she reminded her audience that Florence Nightingale laid the foundations of modern nursing but that her research-mindedness was not passed on as part of the Nightingale tradition. Rather nurses were taught obedience – to superior nurses and, above all, to doctors. Obedience became a virture; critical faculties were to be kept in the background. The idea of a nurse using research methods to examine nursing problems is alien, even today, to many people in our society, to nurses, to doctors, to the public (Simpson, 1971, p. 233). This point will be referred to later in this chapter.

The impetus for nursing research came from various sources: America, where nursing was developing within higher education following the Second World War; changing social circumstances; less rigidity within nursing education and advances in medical practice have all contributed to the need for changes in nursing practice. It was not until 1972 that one of the threads of our cloth became evident. The battle cry 'Nursing must become a research-based profession' began to penetrate the conscious-ness of more than a tiny minority of nurses. The statement comes from the Briggs Report (Report of the Committee on Nursing, 1972) but earlier commentators had made the point. Brotherston (1960), for example, noted that while a minority of any profession might carry out research 'an urgent and understanding sense of the need for research should be a part of the mental equipment of EVERY member of any profession worthy of the name'.

In the previous year, the case was made for a Nursing Research Council (Ouseley, 1959). The author, a lecturer in education at Battersea College, drew attention to the professions of medicine and teaching. The former had (and still has) the Medical Research Council. The teaching profession conducted research through its professional organizations, Local Education Authorities, through its relationships with higher education, as well as the National Foundation for Educational Research. Ouseley believed the time was right to set up a body to look exclusively at nursing research but it seems he was wrong. Apart from the lack of support for his view we should note that both he and Brotherston were from other professions. Later in this chapter we see evidence that the nursing profession has been particularly resistant to change, but has also given the impression that it could, and would, put its own house in order.

A review of the category 'nursing research' in the RCN Bibliography of Nursing (Thompson, 1968, 1974) tells us that in the first 100 years of nursing literature only 83 titles were about nursing research. Only five of them are from the United Kingdom. Two are subjective descriptions of nurses' experience in research teams; one measures the amount of walking done by nurses on the ward. Another studied a nurse tutor course but the work is insufficiently rigorous to be included in the Steinberg Collection of Nursing Research (Lahiff, 1982).*

Among other authors who have written about the development of research in nursing, two have been selected to introduce readers to the topic. Lelean and Clarke (1990) wrote a comprehensive paper on the research resource development, drawing attention to much of the history. They note that during the 15 years from 1953 to 1972, 'research activity was sporadic and focused upon a few individual pioneering nurses such as Norton (1957) and Hockey (1966, 1968)'.

Lelean and Clarke go on to describe the role of government health departments, the National Health Service, the role of professional organiza-tions, nursing statutory bodies, and of higher education. The impression

---

* The Steinberg Collection of Nursing Research is held at the Royal College of Nursing Library, 20 Cavendish Square, London W1M 0AB.

given by that account is one of a fairly smooth, positive series of developments. But it pays little heed to the great challenges of changing the culture
of the profession, of the occupations with which nurses work, or the
organizational structures within which they function.

The second choice is Hockey's *Nursing Research: Mistakes and Misconceptions* (1985). This light-hearted account of things that did or could go wrong
is very accessible and is almost certainly a great help to novice researchers.
But the picture it represents is one all too familiar in nursing: learning by
trial and error. While eventually effective, resources are wasted and damage
is done – to the individual and to respondents; it shows that all too easily a
project can be invalidated through ignorance.

Simpson, Hockey, Lelean and Clarke all pioneered nursing research in
practice, from positions in government and NHS departments, and in
higher education. Simpson describes the framework within which nursing
research was developed. There were three aspects: building up a coherent
research programme, preparing nurses for research, and encouraging the
dissemination and use of research findings. The research programme aimed
to develop research into service, education and practice in all branches of
nursing – hospital, community, GP services – encompassing people of all
ages, and into promoting health, and caring for special groups such as the
physically and mentally ill and handicapped. It was recognized that the
work needed to evolve from descriptive studies into experimentation and
evaluation, together with field trials.

Simpson took up a post in 1963 facing the challenge of bringing a
population of 300 000 trained, employed nurses with little or no knowledge
of nursing research toward becoming a research-based profession. Three
issues were addressed:

1   preparing nurses to carry out research
2   development of research centres
3   dissemination of research findings.

Initiatives to enact the policies included short research-appreciation
courses, the appointment of nursing research liaison officers to each of 14
regions, the institution of a research fellowship scheme, certificated courses
and distance learning opportunities.

Research resource centres were established in Edinburgh (1971), Chelsea
(1977) (now King's College, University of London), and Northwick Park
(1979) (subsequently transferred to the University of Surrey in 1985). These
centres pursued research programmes rather than individual studies and
are still in existence. With the increasing number of academic nursing
departments, research activities are considerably more extensive than when
these initial units began but they remain important contributors. For
example Edinburgh's 40-year-old Department of Nursing Studies was rated
among the top five nursing departments in the UK in the Research

Assessment Exercise, confirming it as one of Britain's foremost research institutions (Tierney, 1996).

Research findings were disseminated with the creation of the Index of Nursing Research in 1976, and the quarterly publication *Nursing Research Abstracts* in 1978. These resources can now be accessed by computer.

Another thread in our canvas was the key initiative by the Royal College of Nursing (RCN). *The Study of Nursing Care* project lasted from 1972 to 1982, and the DHSS underwrote publication of the ensuing monographs at a time when commercial publishers would not consider accepting such material. The 12 studies, covering a range of nursing activities in hospitals and community settings, were analysed by Inman (1975). The theories and contributing sciences used included anxiety, learning, child care, role, communications, stress impairment and the sciences of physiology, psychology, nutrition and biochemistry (McFarlane, 1976). This list gives a good indication of the complexity of nursing, and therefore of the challenges facing the researcher.

McFarlane, another leader in this field, gives an indication of the difficulties she faced when heading up *The Proper Study of the Nurse* project. In an interview with Alison Dunn she states:

> In those early days of the RCN project, I touted round all the universities in the London area to find places where our research assistants could register to do a higher degree. The resistance was terrible. The usual reply was that they couldn't supervise the course because it related to nothing else in the university. (Dunn, 1974)

This problem was overcome serendipitously by meeting the head of the biological sicences department of Surrey University at a reception. This new university had grown out of Battersea College of Advanced Technology, with its history of health-visiting and sister tutor courses.

Another source gives a flavour of the ambivalence felt within the profession at forging links with universities – an essential ingredient if research was to become a reality. In 1947 the RCN made a bold announcement in a national newspaper; *The Times*, that it would, if possible, set up a school to provide undergraduate and postgraduate nursing education. An advisory board was set up but by 1962 it was disbanded having, according to Reinkemeyer, 'withered on the vine' (Reinkemeyer, 1966). The author, whose work will be explored later, comments that this intention may have been the profession's attempt to indicate that it could solve its own problems.

Some observers, then, are less sanguine about the process by which nursing has developed its research activities. But the optimism of pioneers is probably justified when considering their struggles. Simpson concludes that the omens are good, that nurses have found help and encouragement from experienced research workers in a wide range of disciplines and from some nurses in senior positions. Norton states that her view of the development of nursing research is immensely pleasing. Lelean and Clarke declare their optimism about the future of nursing research. 'We believe that there is now a firm foundation for development in this country and that nursing research will certainly "come of age" in the twenty-first century' (Lelean and Clarke, 1990).

So why have nurse researchers had such a difficult time finding secure employment, getting funding, being accepted by other nurses and health professionals? To explore some of these questions we need to examine some very different strands of our history.

The organization of health care

To understand more about nursing and research into its practice we need to explore the setting of agendas: who controls them, and why in the past nursing has apparently had limited success in this area. Key studies are used to explore issues of status, the sexual division of health care together with sex-role stereotyping, concluding with a classic study into the organization of a particular hospital nursing service.

In the past, health care work has been divided into predominently male and female roles, whether occupied by men or women. Professional roots reflected the Victorian context in which they grew. Victorian society was divided rigidly by gender and class. Doctors were originally male – the battle for women to enter the medical profession has already been mentioned. Nursing was exclusively female: for Nightingale a good nurse was a good woman. There is evidence to suggest that she believed women should have educational and vocational opportunities equal to men, and that the nursing profession would provide women with such opportunities (Glass and Brand, 1979). What actually happened was 'the reproduction of the Victorian class structure in the hospital, based on the division of labour between the sexes, and between women of different classes' (Carpenter, 1977, p. 168). Carpenter compares the power and functions of the matron with that of an upper middle-class woman running a Victorian home, where the supreme authority she had over the servants 'complemented but did not subvert the authority of her husband' (p. 168).

Gamarnikow's detailed account of how the nursing role was dictated by the medical profession concludes that:

> Nursing is a unique non-industrial female occupation. It was established and designed for women, and located within a labour process – health care – already dominated by doctors, all of whom were men. Success depended on both creating paid jobs for women who needed them and situating and defining these jobs in a way which would pose no threat to medical authority. The particular form of the sexual division of labour which resulted from this conjuncture is specific to nursing: it is vivid and precise ... emphasis was

placed on the interconnections between femininity, motherhood, housekeeping and nursing. (Gamarnikow, 1978, p. 121)

As all relationships occur within the social order or structure in which they are set, looking at the organization as a whole as well as relationships within it is important. In particular, studying the roles and relationships of groups and subgroups within health care settings reveals valuable insights. Between doctors and nurses Stein revealed a game (Stein, 1968). He argued that doctors needed to appear infallible to patients and nurses, but that they also needed the advice nurses were able to give them. The need to be infallible was seen to arise out of a mixture of the life and death nature of doctor's work, sex-role stereotyping, and their own need to maintain superior status. Both nurse and doctor contributed to the resolution of the dilemma. The nurse gave hints and non-verbal signals to present her advice, sustaining the myth that the doctor alone determined treatment, while he drew on the greater experience the nurse had of the patient, thus hiding her/his contribution to the decision.

While this study is now quite old it is relevent to this exploration because it gives a flavour of organizational relationships. Hockey (1981) describes the changes she has seen in medical attitudes towards nursing research. She stated that in 1962 she recorded the following view: 'No, I have no time for nurses dabbling in research; I have never heard of such nonsense; I won't let them get near my patients' (p. 46). Accepting that there might be a few antagonists around still she went on to say that at the time of writing, the medical profession was more supportive of nursing research, with degrees of support ranging from tolerance to enthusiasm. Her most positive example described an orthopaedic consultant who wanted to work collaboratively with a nurse researcher, recognizing a need for nursing expertise because the nursing of patients (with a fracture of the neck of the femur) was crucial.

Although much has changed, a recent editorial stated 'The doctor–nurse game just won't go away.' In this instance there was more evidence of rivalry than collusion. In a debate about doctor's and nurse's roles the editor points out that the playing field is not level – vast gulfs of class, gender and culture exist, even if they are narrowing. Both professions can be defensive, albeit for differing reasons (Salvage, 1996).

To return to history: besides the relationship with doctors, nurses were also apparently stuck in a social structure which profoundly affected their behaviour. In a classic study of hospital nursing, Menzies (1960) described a profession which avoided change. Senior nursing staff were seeking new methods to organize nursing. They were having increasing difficulty reconciling staffing and training needs, creating acute distress for themselves although they were attempting to raise the status of the nurse as student. At the same time they had to cope with the demands of maintaining appropriate staffing levels to meet patient-care needs. Menzies noted that the existing method of staff allocation had persisted for a long time, without effective modification in spite of its inefficiency. As the study progressed, high levels of tension, distress and anxiety were seen among the nurses. There was much evidence to demonstrate that the levels were beyond tolerating. High sickness rates, withdrawal from training and frequent job changes were all noted. Understanding the anxiety became a key to understanding the development of effective techniques for student–nurse allocation.

Menzies' description of the reality of nursing work remains a classic and is quoted here in full for that reason.

> The situations likely to evoke stress in nurses are familiar. Nurses are in constant contact with people who are physically ill or injured, often seriously. The recovery of patients is not certain and will not always be complete. Nursing patients who have incurable diseases is one of the nurse's most distressing tasks. Nurses are confronted with the threat and the reality of suffering and death as few lay people are. Their work involves carrying out tasks which, by ordinary standards, are distasteful, disgusting, and frightening. Intimate physical contact with patients arouses strong libidinal and erotic wishes and impulses that may be difficult to control. The work situation arouses very strong and mixed feelings in the nurse: pity, compassion, and love; guilt and anxiety; hatred and resentment of the patient who arouses these strong feelings; envy of the care given to the patient. (Menzies, 1960, 1970, p. 5)

To manage these deep, confused, subconscious feelings, Menzies described a set of defensive techniques in the nursing service, several of which are particularly relevant to our investigation of why nursing research has taken so long to be included as part of the nurse's world. These are:

- the attempt to eliminate decisions by ritual task-performance
- reducing the weight of responsibility in decision-making by checks and counter-checks
- purposeful obscurity in the formal distribution of responsibility
- the reduction of the impact of responsibility by delegation to superiors
- idealization and underestimation of personal development possibilities
- avoidance of change.

Space precludes sharing all the evidence brought to underpin this list, but a few examples give a flavour of how relevant this work is. In ritual task-performance, Menzies states that: 'Making a decision implies making a choice between possible courses of action and committing oneself to one of them; the choice being made in the absence of full factual information' (p. 15). To spare staff the resulting anxiety, the nursing service attempted to minimize the number and variety of decisions to be made by giving precise instructions about the way a task was to be performed, in what order and at which time. Where several efficient methods for a task existed, one was chosen and performed exclusively. A lot of effort was expended on standardizing nursing procedures – turning tasks into 'rituals'. All work was treated with almost life and death seriousness and student nurses were actively discouraged from using their own discretion and initiative. Similar constraints were applied to senior staff, although with more difficulty.

The defense mechanism 'collusive social redistribution of responsibility and irresponsibility' was seen to arise from the attempt to resolve the painful responsibility of the nurse's role. As this was difficult to bear consistently, nurses were tempted to give it up. To deal with the intra-psychic conflict, at least in part, it was converted into an interpersonal conflict by describing certain nurses as responsible and others as irrespons-ible. Often whole categories of nurses would be classified in this way; usually junior nurses were seen as less responsible than the person describ-ing them.

The researchers came to realize that the complaints were the result of a collusive system of denial, splitting off and projecting what is undesirable within oneself on to others. Not only was this seen as culturally acceptable to nurses, it was required of them. The roles assigned to senior and junior nurses – the one as harsh disciplinarians and the others as irresponsible – were what they became.

Finally, a look at 'the reduction of the impact of responsibility by delegation to superiors'. Apparently the word 'delegation' used in the hospital being studied seemed to mean the opposite to its meaning else-where. In ordinary use it implies that a superior hands over a task, and the responsibility for it, to a subordinate. In this case, however, tasks were often forced upwards into the hierarchy, and responsibility for them disclaimed. This effectively reduces the burden of responsibility on the person con-cerned. The research team were struck by the low level of tasks carried out by nurses in relation to their personal ability, skill and official position. People at quite senior levels were told what to do. In particular, the task of assigning students to wards was done by assistant matrons.

Menzies and her team could see that given a clearly defined policy this task could have been performed efficiently by a competent clerk. They perceived that subordinate nurses felt very dependent on their superiors, expecting them to make decisions for them, while nurses as superiors felt unable to trust their juniors. Plans to change things for the better were received enthusiastically at first but as lower-level staff began to identify the decisions they would have to make, they requested the seniors to continue as before. The overburdened senior staff apparently accepted the task willingly.

Whether these findings were intrinsic to the type of work nursing is about, as Menzies argued, or are related to the relationship with medicine, or are more characteristic of hierarchical organizations is questionable. They could also be related to the fact that, at that time, most nursing work was carried out by partly trained student nurses with an inadequate knowledge-base from which to make good decisions.

Menzies' research may seem a far cry from the current situation, when many aspects of health service organization and the nursing service within it have changed almost beyond recognition. But it helps our understanding of why the agenda for nursing research has been set and actioned slowly, both by nurse leaders and clinical practitioners. Issues of responsibility are central to becoming research-minded. If the culture of nursing has a long history of being denied responsibility by doctors, and of nurses being perceived as irresponsible by their senior colleagues, it is unlikely that they could change swiftly into questioning their practice and looking for valida-tion of existing practice, or new and better ways of meeting patients' and clients' needs.

In her concluding comments, Menzies describes the nursing service as having acute anxieties combined with a series of defence mechanisms which were primitive and ineffectual. Giving up known ways of behaving to embark on the unknown seemed to be intolerable, with the threat of social chaos and individual breakdown. In the hospital being studied, while the senior staff discussed the proposals made to change and improve the situation they had asked for help with, they felt unable to proceed with the plans to do so.

It seemed likely that what the researchers experienced at this one hospital was fairly typical of similar general nurse training schools at the time. Menzies writes that few professions have been more studied than nursing, or institutions more studied than hospitals. In many instances nurses initiated or willingly took part in these studies. They saw that nursing faced crucial changes, eagerly sought solutions, but 'one is astonished to find how little basic or dynamic change has taken place. Nurses have tended to receive reports and recommendations with a sense of outrage and to react to them by intensifying current attitudes and reinforcing existing practice' (Menzies 1960, 1970, p. 41).

The issues around nursing relationships which have been explored briefly here can be studied in greater depth elsewhere. Heyman and Shaw (1984) worked on the subject for some years. They commented that attempts to make British nurse training more orientated to the improve-ment of communications were oversimplistic. The gap which arose between the ideals taught in school and the reality of ward practice was likely to be great. They saw a number of factors involved: the distribution of inter-professional power, the bureaucratic organization, the influence of different social statuses such as class and gender, combined with a cultural ambi-valence towards sickness and death.

A similar situation exists with nursing research. Teaching nursing stu-dents to read research reports, to question those who teach them in practice, is to oversimplify the reality. Nurses who were conditioned early in their work to obey doctors and seniors, to play a game with doctors which denied their own contribution to patient care, and which disseminated responsibility away from themselves, were likely to have difficulty with the notion of professional responsibility – which is a necessary precursor to valuing research.

The place of education in research

A widely held view both within (and outside) nursing has been that education will deliver the changes which were seen as desirable by nurse leaders, whether to provide a leadership pool, nurses educated to undertake research, or product champions to help change nursing practice. Such an approach avoided tackling the organization within which nursing actually took place; it also maintained the *status quo*.

In her paper 'The development of degree courses in nursing education – in historical and professional context' Owen (1984) describes five phases of progress, beginning with the Nightingale era. The second phase – the struggle for registration, state examinations and the creation of a statutory body – took place between 1900 and 1925. A period of consolidation followed until the 1948 Nurses Act allowed for experimental courses in basic nurse training to take place, which opened up the way for collaboration with higher education. From the 1950s onwards, a gradual evolution of degree courses began. The paper concentrates on the fifth phase: collaboration with higher education and basic nurse education. But what of the earlier phases?

Early in the development of the nursing profession two key leaders emerged. One is well known – Nightingale. The other, Ethel Bedford-Fenwick, is known mainly to nurses who have studied their professional history. The one became a national heroine; the other, who was a key figure in the politics of nursing, is unknown to the public at large.

Mrs Fenwick had been matron at St Bartholomew's Hospital in the 1880s, resigning her position when she married. Described as a 'restless genius' she differed from Nightingale in several respects – not least because she campaigned for nurses to be registered (McGann, 1992). She also believed that nurses should have access to higher education and was instrumental in the establishment of a Diploma in Nursing in the Extra-Mural Department of London University in the early years of the century. This course was available mainly on a part-time basis for more than 70 years. As in many other areas, curriculum and examinations were controlled by the medical profession. But as nurses took charge of their own agenda they assumed control, designing and implementing a new curriculum in the 1980s.

The revised curriculum, with its unit structure, introduced nurses to research, many of them for the first time. It helped them read and interpret research findings, and required the submission of in-depth nursing studies which drew on research findings to underpin their practice.

Teaching research on this course met, in some instances, with hostility. Subsequently, however, nurses appreciated the richness of research findings as they were called on to deal with more complex patient-care issues, many of which were the outcome of advances in medical practice and technology.

Courses (to prepare nurse tutors and health visitors) were based, in some instances, in higher education. Although they had been there for several decades, they do not appear to have been greatly influenced by the ethos of education. The first health visitor to undertake research came into nursing as a graduate (Clark, 1973). The Council for the Education and Training of Health Visitors, founded in 1964, took ten years to publish the first piece of work it commissioned (Gilmore, Bruce and Hunt, 1974).

Research appreciation was put into the tutor's course at some stage; according to an interviewee in research conducted by the author:

> the tutors nearly went up in smoke because they knew nothing about research – and they've got this idea that it's something which they can't get to grips with – that it is very high-powered and terribly academic. (Lahiff, 1982, p. 38)

In that study only one person reported being introduced to nursing research during her basic SRN training in 1975–78. Other members of the group had first met with it when studying for degree or diploma courses; one had discovered it while a ward sister and two others had been research assistants to doctors.

As stated earlier, experimental basic nurse training courses became possible in 1948. The existing links with higher education were not exploited until 1957 when four courses were established in institutions with nursing association. Called integrated courses, they linked traditional nurse education with higher education. Students acquired nurse registration, health visiting and, in some cases, district nursing certificates. Although the entrance requirement was equivalent to university entrance, the courses were all at certificate level for some years. Later these courses evolved into degrees, the first one at Manchester in the mid-1960s. Issues around this development will be discussed below.

Eventually other institutions followed but even so all these developments had only very small student numbers compared to traditional courses. With the exception of Manchester, they all focused on basic nurse education. The need to offer undergraduate courses to qualified nurses developed several years later with part-time nursing degrees becoming available from 1980. Until then Manchester's Diploma in Advanced Nursing which could lead to a Master's degree, and the University of London's Diploma, were the only post-basic academic courses in clinical nursing.

To establish which educational agendas were being set and by whom, we need to consider what the lead bodies in nursing were doing at this time. Mention of has already been made of the RCN's 1947 statement of intent to link with a university – but their procrastination led Reinkemeyer (1966) to describe it as a paralysing do-nothing policy.

The General Nursing Council for England and Wales set up a research unit in 1967. Funded by the Ministry of Health for five years it was greeted enthusiastically by the Editor of the Nursing Times:

> Everyone will rejoice that the General Nursing Council for England and Wales is to establish its own research unit. There must be a mass of material in the files awaiting documentation, analysis and publication, upon which action can be taken.

and later:

> We are less happy that the GNC has succumbed to the current gimmickry for 'evaluation'; it was said at the press conference that the research unit would be undertaking 'evaluation of experimental schemes'. We have, on a previous occasion, pointed out the difficulties, if not the impossibility of such an excercise. What are the criteria? (*Nursing Times*, Editorial, 1967)

Simpson pointed out in her review of the first steps in nursing research that education had been most frequently studied from the point of view of recruitment, selection and withdrawal of student – over 70 studies at that time (Simpson, 1971, p. 25). Reviewing the studies, Simpson highlights many problems: the studies are small-scale and inconclusive, descriptive, lacking in theoretical frameworks.

Another study aimed to establish the number of graduates among practising nurses. Although it had been noted in 1956 that this information would be useful, neither the GNC nor the MoH had decided to collect it (MacGuire, 1970). It was estimated that 60 nurses had degrees in 1953; by 1970 the number was 483. The articles in which the figures appeared gave little indication of how to use the information.

The GNC published some of its findings – MacGuire's (1969) *Threshold to Nursing* is an example. But a history of the GNC 1919–1969 makes no mention of research or experimental programmes (Bendall and Raybould, 1969). It appears to be yet another descriptive study which gives little indication that this body was setting an agenda related to higher education or nursing research.

Paradoxically it was around this time that the DHSS was taking a lead in the development of nurse researchers. Lelean and Clarke (1990) outline the initiatives which included fellowships to prepare people at Master's level for research work, and assistance for others to complete first degrees. But against a work force of 300 000 the numbers were miniscule. The original plan to assist 12 people to complete first degrees dropped to eight in the early 1980s and disappeared within a few years as educational opportunities in nursing increased.

As with pre-registration developments, the opening up of poor registration educational programmes was more to do with individual leadership and organizational opportunities than any specific professional leadership initiatives. The author's experiences of developing such a programme were a mixture of highs and lows. Highs because the students were so exciting, committed and a joy to work with; lows because of the opposition from senior nurses who did not believe that clinical nursing was worth studying, coupled with hostility from students' colleagues in some cases (Lahiff, 1984). Both staff and students were told that only management or education was worth studying at degree level. This particular course focused on clinical practice – a rare philosophy at that time.

On the other side of the Atlantic an American nurse, Agnes Reinkemeyer, was aware of the divisions between hospital- and university-trained nurses. She noted the hostility towards higher education for nurses and the difficulties of getting research findings into practice. She decided to study the first such developments in the United Kingdom (Reinkemeyer, 1966). Much of what follows here is drawn from her doctoral thesis.

Reinkemeyer revealed that the British experimental programmes of nurse education were the end-products of 50 years of professional conflict. Discontent with the deficiencies in traditional nurse training were over-shadowed by resistance to change. The idea of nursing education being located in universities was deplored. The key reason given for developing the courses was to attract students with university entrance to be the leadership pool of the future.

By interviewing nurse leaders, such as hospital matrons, nursing tutors, nurses in government departments, regional and area nurse managers and nursing journalists (29 in total), Reinkemeyer established that people were looking for immediate benefits for the profession. They seemed to perceive nursing as needing 'saving' and some better-qualified (on entry) nurses would do that. Evidently university association was sought and supported as a 'last resort'. In Reinkemeyer's view, the respondents did not possess firm convictions that there was a need for basic university programmes. Much doubt and fear was expressed as to whether it was the 'right' approach to the profession's problems. The upgrading of entrants was seen as the only way to attract people of high intellectual ability and to retain them. One matron observed that, with more girls (!) going to university it would be necessary to take 'the second and third cream rather than the first' (p. 362).

Respondents had clear views that entrants with university backgrounds would become, in due course, the leaders able to take the administrative and teaching posts. But two other points were made: 'saving face *vis-à-vis* other professions' and 'maintaining international eminence' (p. 363). Reinkemeyer considered that:

in the final analysis, it seemed that the slight impact the 'experimental' graduates promised to make on British nursing as a whole could be traced to the non-stimulating, constricted and rejecting climate of the present education-ally deprived nursing profession. (p. 495)

According to Reinkemeyer's informants, British nurses were the best in the world. They apparently rejected any notion that nursing practice might need evaluating, in much the same way as evaluating experimental courses was rejected by a nursing journal editor. And nurses were not alone in their view of themselves: it was a line taken by hospital boards and many doctors despite the fact that many others were expressing the view that 'the condition of nursing is deplorable' (p. 112).

Three fundamental and interrelated factors appeared to underline the nurse leaders' hesitancy about moving into higher education:

1 they did not WANT university courses for what the university had to give, namely intellectual development of students.
2 they DENIED that nursing could be an academic subject or REFUSED to come to grips with the implications of that proposition.
3 they were UNWILLING to admit that the university should control the nursing course, or were disinclined to deal with what such an admission would mean.
(Hubert/Reinkemeyer, 1967)

Like Menzies, Reinkemeyer reached some unpalatable conclusions which did not endear her to British nurses. She considered that both they and her American compatriots had a marked anti-intellectualism – a paradox where there was a simultaneous demand for and rejection of university-based programmes and their graduates. In Britain, nurses were seen to resist any notion that nursing practice needed to be changed. Leaders in professional organizations took an ultra-conservative position, paying lip service to the notion of change while failing to make decisive moves in that direction.

A 'paralysing ambivalence' was how Reinkemeyer described what she perceived.

> With rare exception British nurses were found to be indifferent, confused, or openly hostile regarding demands for university-based programmes. To vindicate their negative positions they gradually built up a network of psychosocial defences which rendered the profession ever more resistant to educational development. Myths, rationalisations and taboos were adduced to prove that nurses only needed dedication and not education. A fascinating confusion of Victorian religious, moralistic, and social class notions – these inventions continue to inhibit educational progress today. (Hubert/Reinkemeyer, 1967)

So here we have another significant study which demonstrates the profession's ambivalence towards change: apparently wanting to set new agendas but somehow sabotaging the effort even before any real change took place.

It is difficult to find satisfactory explanations of what was happening. As Menzies had identified, nurses saw problems, recognized the need for change, but then rejected or only half-heartedly supported new approaches. Having recognized the need for a new agenda, they then qualified it by demanding that graduate nurses be as good as traditionally trained ones. That they might be better was not considered.

Could it be a problem of self-image, as the following passage suggests?

Women and nurses have not systematically learned to value themselves. In this male-dominated society, females learn to care for others rather than themselves and as a result have not nurtured their own self-images. Adult women are faced with the incongruity of being expected to perform professionally and autonomously but at the same time to play the traditionally feminine, passive role. This incongruity leads to stress upon the self-concept of women and nurses. (Bush and Kjervick, 1979)

Only fragments of Reinkemeyer's thesis have been referred to here. Among many omissions is the tribute she paid to the individuals who developed these experimental programmes. Using different approaches to problems they each identified, they faced up to the difficulties of solving them in the absence of any systematic planning or unified effort on the part of the British nursing profession. The fact remains that these pioneers went down a path which, even 40 years later, as nursing takes its place in higher education, still has vociferous opponents.

The development of nurse researchers and clinical practice

Earlier in this chapter we saw something of the views of pioneers in nursing research. Norton pointed out that 30 years ago there was no academic (nursing) world to have views about! Later she said that there was a tendency for a minority group of nurse researchers to take on an air of superiority in the eyes of the majority. As a Regional Nurse Research Liaison Officer she often had to defend the role of the research entrepreneur. There was a view that research was seen as a vehicle of academic progress rather than to serve the practice of nursing (Norton, 1985).

Various examples give some indication of the climate in which these pioneers worked. Hockey (1985, p. 2) describes some of the obstacles to her questions as far back as the Second World War: 'At that time it seemed that nothing could be done to get answers to simple questions.' In my general nursing training days in the 1950s, a psychology graduate left in her second year because she was discouraged from asking questions – a difficulty not understood by her peers. 'If you want to be loved, stay away from research,' stated a speaker at a research conference in the 1980s. He went on to point out that researchers have never been popular because they ask too many questions, and people like a quiet life (Payne, 1983).

In the early 1980s a survey of nurse researchers highlighted some of the difficulties they faced (Lahiff, 1982). Structured interviews, conducted with a dozen people, identified a group of people relatively isolated from colleagues in clinical practice and often viewed with suspicion by them. Their routes into research were diverse and unpredicted, their status unclear and, in some instances, their future career prospects were far from certain.

The majority of the group were graduates, having entered higher education following their nurse training. All but one of the non-graduates was registered for a degree – which indicates their recognition of the necessity for post-basic graduate education for undertaking research work.

As most of the group were studying patient-care topics, the difficulties of doing so were explored. For example, the proposition was put to each of them that the topics chosen avoided conflict with the medical profession was accepted.

> There's a lot more potential (in the 'Cinderella areas') for the nurse to do something about it – less fighting – and because these are areas which lend themselves to nursing change.

> nurses have always been able to take over things once medics have been bored with them.

> Yes – my research was in a 'Cinderella area' – and the conflict isn't as pertinent as it would be in an acute area – if you tried to do something where a surgeon has very definite ideas – we are doing something now in pain control and that's the anaesthetist's province – so any change we try to make with that will be a much more multidisciplinary area. (Lahiff, 1982, p. 23)

The term 'Cinderella areas' seems to be used here to describe health care activities which are either clearly the work of the nurse, such as pressure area management and incontinence, or an area like communication. The latter is seen as more compatable with the nurse's role as 'carer'. They were also topics which were considered to lend themselves to nursing change; they were poorly catered for at that time, and the power that came from having research evidence was needed. Here we have examples of nurses setting their own agenda, albeit in a way which bypassed overt conflict with the medical profession and which made sense in the developmental stages of becoming a research-based profession.

The strategy of conflict avoidance could not always be relied on. One respondent, having chosen a nursing topic, discovered that there were important implications for medical treatment. She said:

> There are doctors who are interested in the problem I have uncovered, and they are happy to fight for nurses ... but they are not so happy to have their clinical judgement challenged. We shall have to come to some sort of compromise. (Lahiff, 1982, p. 23)

As we shall see later, some nurses found that diplomatic skills were necessary to avoid conflict.

Despite setting agendas, nurses still had to run the gauntlet of ethical committees and research-funding bodies. These were dominated by doctors, most of whom had limited knowledge of research methodologies other than the clinical trial. A nurse member of one such committee said she felt as if nurses were being allowed to 'play at' doing research.

Anything that sniffs of sociology, or includes a questionnaire ... they will nit pick ... Because nursing research has a sociological basis – a lot of it – it's not seen as very credible. (Lahiff, 1982, p. 25)

However, some changes were noted: an initially doubtful consultant on a multidisciplinary research committee read all the papers, attended all the meetings, and eventually became an ally who gained the cooperation of other consultants, thus enabling other nurses to undertake research.

Apart from the difficulties of choosing a topic area which would avoid conflict, and getting the approval of ethics committees, control was exercised through funding with committees at central, regional and local level dominated by doctors. Several individuals clearly had good personal relationships with medical colleagues and reported no conflicts. But the management of relationships was recognized as important.

I don't threaten them (the doctors) in any way – I'm actually very careful about upsetting people – although I know exactly what I want – I think this is where the diplomacy comes in because you don't achieve anything at the end of the day, especially if they are in a more powerful position – which they are. (Lahiff, 1982, p. 26)

Turning to the issue of implementing research findings, several people reported interest in and acceptance of their work by ward-based nurses. Others considered that the attitudes of senior nurse managers and tutors were important, together with the need for findings to be more comprehensible to the ordinary nurse.

In general, respondents in the survey were optimistic about nurses wanting research findings:

The reluctance is higher up the scale ... not with grass-root level. Once their eyes are opened through research ... and I ask so many questions – they begin to question things themselves.

I think a lot of nurses are very willing to be presented with new information – relevant stuff which will help them with their care.

One of the most rewarding things about my job is that somebody actually wants me to do research and they want the results and they are now prepared to take the consequences, whereas a few years ago if I said something, it was ... 'Who's she?' – whereas that has changed to some extent. (Lahiff, 1982, p. 43)

Not everyone had such positive views, particularly those with experience in North America.

In the States nursing research is valued much more highly than here ... a professional nurse with a degree has acquired the sorts of skills associated with being a good consumer of research.

They (American nurses) are much more well-informed about things that nurses in this country don't necessarily seek an awareness of – like research – they are much more research-orientated. (Lahiff, 1982, p. 44)

The effect of becoming a researcher on individual careers produced some interesting, and at times unexpected, responses. For a start these nurses, like many others, entered nursing with no career strategy or expectations. Several people found their basic nurse training was intellectually dissatisfying; three of them made plans to go to university while still in training. The responses of their superiors confirm Reinkemeyer's findings. While one matron was encouraging, others were not. A Director of Nurse Education refused to give a reference for the UCCA form, stating that a university education was totally unnecessary. These experiences, which cover the mid-1960s to the mid-1970s, were coupled with a belief that the individuals concerned would not return to nursing.

Re-entry into the profession had its problems, some of which were resolved by the introduction of nurse-research fellowships and other opportunities to undertake research. The profession seemed to have difficulties assimilating this new activity in its ranks.

I can tell you it's not very comfortable, this sort of life ... and one really wonders if one has been foolish ... on the other hand there is interest and, to some extent, excitement.

Another respondent identified her ideal job:

I became interested in research and decided my ideal role would be one where I had a clinical component, a research component, but also retained my teaching component. (Lahiff, 1982, p. 41)

For the five respondents holding NHS research posts, their work provided opportunities for them to use their expertise in interesting and pioneering ways. They joined support networks to sustain them in their lonely work; they spoke of isolation, relationship difficulties and antagonism as well as acceptance, cooperation and good relationships. They recognized though that, in meeting with each other, the finger of élitism was pointed at them, and that they should, perhaps, have cultivated better relationships with nurse managers and educators.

In this research three strategies were identified for using research to improve the quality of care: having a nursing research committee to vet nursing research proposals that did not affect medical treatment; getting the right credentials for doing research; and finally diplomacy. Combined with the loneliness and, for some, the alienation, being a nurse researcher was a challenging experience but one which all the respondents appeared to enjoy. Many of them have gone on to exercise major leadership roles in nursing and health care today. Presumably the lessons they learned in setting nursing research agendas two decades ago are being used to good effect now that clinical effectiveness is a key agenda item within the health service.

The picture in the 1990s is very different. Whereas research findings could only be found in specialist journals, now the weekly nursing publications draw heavily on research findings and include regular research updates. Critical reviews of research findings, such as those published by the NHS Centre for Reviews and Dissemination, bring together the knowledge available to underpin practice.

The Centre has a particular remit to address nursing and is facilitating the establishment of regional databases so that nurses can quickly establish what work has been done or is being undertaken in a particular area (O'Meara and Dickson, 1996). By networking, the individuals and groups concerned can avoid the duplication of effort and make maximum use of scarce resources. While there are some legitimate concerns about the limitations of the clinical effectiveness philosophy, it is a far cry from the situation research pioneers found themselves in two and three decades ago.

All the years of preparation, of developing research awareness, skills and knowledge, through a battery of increased education opportunities at different levels, and against a traditional mind-set which represented barren soil in which early ideas had to struggle to take root, are bearing fruit today. As databases are established throughout the country, based on rigorous appraisal of nursing research findings, nursing research is coming of age.

There are many examples now to indicate how far nurses have travelled to become a research-based profession. The growth in the number of academic nursing departments, the accessibility of research findings in a range of weekly and monthly nursing journals, the numbers of research papers being presented at the many national and international nursing conferences, all contribute their evidence. Like the pioneers it is possible to be positive about the future for nursing research, given that it will always have difficulties, in common with other disciplines. Having a brief look at the past, however, demonstrates how much has depended on individual rather than collective agenda-setting until the last decade or so.

Power, autonomy and control

To get to grips with the gap between rhetoric and reality, between the policies of nurses at government level and the reality of nurses' work, and the effect of organizational relationships on nurses and research, it is important to explore issues of power and control – essential assets in setting research agendas.

We will start with a simple premise: that in the past there was little point in the individual nurse in clinical practice questioning what was done, in the absence of having the power to change anything. This key issue needs to be understood when exploring the challenges facing the nursing profession, whether at national level, getting resources to prepare researchers and to fund research, or at the clinical level where nurses want to implement research findings.

Few occupations are so closely related as nursing and medicine. Neither can function fully without the other, except in fairly limited situations. To ensure that patients and clients receive the best care, each needs the other to be well-prepared for their work. Ideally, nurses and doctors should work together as collaborating equals, respecting each other's skills and expertise. While there are instances where this happens, for the most part the reality is very different, and in the past nurses were clearly subservient to doctors.

To a large extent health care issues are often unclear because medicine is considered to be the sole focus; in the media the term 'medicine' is often used as a synonym for health care. Health-related soap operas have the doctor as hero and the nurse as a walk-on part or, all too frequently, providing the love interest. Even documentaries tell us about the miracles of modern surgery with little or no reference to the multitude of other professionals whose skills and expert knowledge contributed to both pre- and post-operative care. Nursing, among other occupations, is usually hidden, or kept in a subsidiary role.

Earlier in this chapter key research reports were used to examine the past. But an alternative method is to revisit historical events with a different set of assumptions. In her book, *Rewriting Nursing History* Davies (1980) illustrated the constraints which prevented nurses from getting what they set out to achieve. She considers that many of the historical events available for study do not have much to say about the often covert conflicts nurses have had with the medical profession.

In another observation Davies considers that dependency and control over others have been hallmarks of nursing (Davies, 1976). This occupational strategy operates for several reasons. Not only has it been a historical legacy, it has also been consonant with feminine values, and it solved problems for individuals and organizations.

Witz (1992), in her account of the battle for nurse registration, considers that the 1919 Nurses Registration Act was not a victory for those nurses in favour of it but a significant defeat. She described Mrs Bedford-Fenwick's campaign for nurse registration as a female professional project. Her vision – of a state-sponsored body in which nurses formed a clear majority – posed a strong challenge to existing sets of power relations. Among her proposals was the separation of nurse education from the staffing needs of hospitals – something only achieved almost 100 years later.

In contrast, Witz argues, the professional project of medicine was facilitated by the ability of medical men to exclude women from their strategy, because civil and state institutions were structured on patriarchal lines. It was therefore possible for the emerging health care professions to be divided on a gender basis. This situation has led, inevitably, to tension in nursing unless it simply accepts a subordinate role. To assert itself as an independent profession, it has to struggle both with itself and with medical colleagues.

Sociological analysis of professions has included requirements such as a distinctive knowledge base, self-governance, autonomy and control over work, combined with elements of service, and the relationship with the client which has been seen as the source of power. Examining the relationships between doctors and nurses centres more recently on power and the struggles over position.

In their study of doctors and nurses, Walby and Greenwell (1994) identified both occupations as having quite different notions of what they meant by the term 'professional'. They found that each considered the other to be non-professional, but neither seemed to notice that the differences existed – thus providing a basis for the tensions they observed in everyday practice.

> The medical notion of a profession was one where an educated person was able to respond to individual problems in undetermined, innovative yet trustworthy ways. The nursing notion was one of technicality, of pinning down exactly what was to be done and the training and staff needed to do it to agreed standards. (p. 61)

The disagreements over whether or not nurses should give intravenous drugs seemed to be tied into these differing perceptions. Doctors considered nurses were able to do things which the latter wanted rules to follow. Conversely, nurses were critical of the lack of control and supervision of junior doctors.

Some of this tension can be explained by lack of knowledge and understanding. Doctors have been shown to believe that nurses have more knowledge than they actually have. Certainly some nurses have, rightly, refused to undertake some doctors' work on the grounds that they lack appropriate knowledge. All too often, though, only the technical aspects of delegated tasks are seen; insufficient attention is paid to the knowledge base required to respond to adverse reactions, for example. As we have already seen, one way of containing anxiety has been to provide rules. The latter system makes sense when much nursing work was (and still is) carried out by untrained or partially trained staff.

Recent research about medicine and nursing poses the question whether doctors and nurses are allies or adversaries (Walby and Greenwell, 1994). The authors state that the positions may be considered simultaneously as both symbiotically related professions and also competitors. As well as occupying positions within the medical division of labour in which they need the work of the other to be carried out effectively, they are also in a hierarchical relationship in which they are each jockeying for position. Walby and Greenwell state:

There has long been a tension in nursing as to whether it accepts a clearly subordinate role to medicine or whether it can assert itself as an independent profession with a less unequal status to medicine. (p. 56)

Wound management is a topic comprehensively researched by nurses, probably because it has constituted a significant part of nursing work. Walby and Greenwell found:

that some doctors would listen to nursing research, others had to be approached 'diplomatically' if nursing staff were to succeed in having their prescription choice agreed, and a small number of doctors flatly refused to look at research papers, or listen to the views of nursing staff. (Walby and Greenwell, 1994, p. 43)

Examining professional boundaries in conjunction with wound management the authors stated:

increasing interest by doctors in wounds may be related to the fact that wound treatment is an area in which there is a development of research. Wound healing is therefore an area of expertise where nurses justify their claim to control care by reference to scientific knowledge and practical experience, precisely the same criteria that medicine uses to justify its status. (p. 42)

The tensions arise not just because the professions are different but because they are interdependent. As nursing moves towards the medical concept of an autonomous individual, and the medical profession, by accepting medical audit, moves towards nursing notions of accountability, the situation can change. The devolution of authority downwards in hospitals is changing the professional authority which is expressed through hierarchical structures. These authors consider that as long as doctors 'own' patients, nurses will remain in subordinate positions. While there is a self-interest in seeing each other improve, conflict is inevitable when it challenges authority.

These tensions can been seen in the many areas where clinical nurse specialists are found. Consultants clearly value and support nurses extending their roles, their knowledge and sphere of influence – as long as the consultants think they 'own' nurses and their work. They are more likely to oppose developments in ward organization, such as primary nursing. They are also, apparently, threatened by nurses using words they would like to own, such as 'practitioner', 'consultant', 'diagnose', 'prescribe', even though these words are used by many other occupational groups in settings far removed from health care.

That nurses have always had authority is not in doubt. The question is whether they can combine it with autonomy. Hunt and Wainwright (1994) quote Bishop and Scudder:

Of course, nurses do not have the authority to make the same decisions that physicians and administrators have, but nurses have their own particular kind of authority. Nurses have the authority and power that comes from the control of day-to-day care of the patient.

The authors suggest that instead of engaging in struggles for professional autonomy, nurses should use the space they have to develop their existing authority and change everyday practices in a piecemeal fashion within the power relations of the *status quo*. Concern with autonomy, they argue, disrupts cooperative teamwork. This perspective connects with one referred to above, about Victorian middle-class women not usurping their husbands' authority overtly, and using such power as they already had to manipulate situations to achieve their objectives.

Hunt and Wainwright conclude that the tensions between the different occupational groups in health care will continue into the future. They postulate differing potential scenarios: that nursing could be submerged and controlled by doctors and accountants, or more positively that nurses seize the moral highground of health care and determine for themselves what skills and tasks are required for the benefit of patients.

Whichever approach is taken – and different situations will call for different solutions – progress will be made as robust research into nursing practices becomes available, as more nurses gain in confidence through better academic preparation, and as they become increasingly assertive and work collectively to achieve their aims.

Conclusion

Using an eclectic approach, this chapter has drawn a personal picture of the development of nursing research in the United Kingdom. Selections from the literature, the views of some nurse-research pioneers and a few key findings about the social context of the profession and the organization in which it has worked have been described. Over several decades the scene has changed from one where individuals created agendas, using local circumstances to advantage but often battling against considerable odds to achieve their ends, and without a coordinated professional drive towards their goals.

As Clay (1987) pointed out nursing has looked, all too often, for a single solution to a multitude of problems. One of the perceived solutions has been research. There is no doubt it can be a powerful tool in getting the best care to patients and clients. But insight into the broader picture can help nurses to be more realistic in understanding why the change process seems to take so long when changes of other kinds happen so quickly.

The leaders of nursing research were right to be optimistic in their backward look at where they had come from, and the journey they had travelled. They took on a professional group ill-equipped for change, able to resist it like few others, defeated in some ways even when they were apparently successful, locked simultaneously into a very difficult symbiotic yet competitive relationship with doctors, in a hierarchical relationship governed largely by the gender roles of 100 years ago. Those who trod the first steps are to be applauded for their acceptance of the loneliness and the struggles. They were inspired by their vision of what could be, and we are the inheritors of that vision. While we have to tailor it to what is possible now, there are signs that some of the changes in health care are weakening the professional authority which was expressed in hierarchical structures and which was so limiting.

It is useful to remind ourselves of Mahler's vision for nursing:

> If millions of nurses in a thousand different places articulate the same ideas and convictions about primary health care and come together as one force then they could act as a powerhouse for change. (WHO Features, WHO, July 1985)

The same is true of nurses using research. Today national and international agendas are being set. Clinical effectiveness is a major theme in the NHS. The International Council of Nurses published *Better Health Through Nursing Research* as the focus for International Nurses Day in 1996. What a contrast to Norton's remarks about an upstairs-downstairs situation: upstairs the research gentry, downstairs the day-to-day problems of patient care and keeping the service going. That may still be visible in some places – but in others research findings are being sought and used downstairs. The current picture is considerably more positive than the one described by the pioneers, despite all the upheavals which continue to take place in health care delivery, and the all-too-familiar constraints.

References

Bendall E R D and Raybould E (1969) *A History of the General Nursing Council for England and Wales 1919–1969*. H K Lewis, London.

Brotherston J H F (1960) Research mindedness and the health professions. In *Learning to Investigate Nursing Problems*. International Council of Nurses and Florence Nightingale International Foundation, London.

Bush M A and Kjervik D K (1979) The nurse's self-image. In Kjervik D K and Martinson I M (1979) *Women in Stress: a Nursing Perspective*. Appleton-Century-Crofts, New York.

Carpenter M (1977) The new managerialism and professionalism in nursing. In Stacey M *et al.* (1977) *Health Care and the Division of Labour*. Croom Helm, London.

Clark J (1973) *A Family Visitor*. Royal College of Nursing, London.

Clay T (1987) *Nurses: Power and Politics*. Heinemann Nursing, London.

Davies C (1976) Experience of dependency and control in work: the case of nurses. *Journal of Advanced Nursing*, I: 273–82.

Davies C (ed.) (1980) *Rewriting Nursing History*. Croom Helm, London.

Dunn A (1974) Research – use and abuse: Jean McFarlane talks to Alison Dunn. *Nursing Times* 70(12) 21 March: 442–3.

Gamarnikow E (1978) Sexual division of labour: the case of nursing. In Kuhn A and Wolfe A (1978) (eds) *Feminism and Materialism*. Routledge and Kegan Paul, London.

Gilmore M, Bruce N and Hunt M (1974) *The Work of the Nursing Team in General Practice.* CETHV, London.

Glass L K and Brand K P (1979) The progress of women and nursing: parallel or divergent? In Kjervik D K and Martinson I M (1979) *Women in Stress: A Nursing Perspective.* Appleton-Century-Croft, New York.

Heyman B and Shaw M (1984) Looking at relationships in nursing. In Skevington S (1984) *Understanding Nurses.* John Wiley, Chichester.

Hockey L (1981) Knowledge is a precious possession. *Nursing Mirror.* 153(13) 23 Sept: 46–9.

Hockey L (1985) *Nursing Research: Mistakes and Misconceptions.* Churchill Livingstone, Edinburgh.

Hubert M (1967) British nursing and the universities: an American view. *Nursing Times* 63(40–46) inclusive.

Hunt G and Wainwright P (1994) *Expanding the Role of the Nurse: the Scope of Professional Practice.* Blackwell Scientific, London.

Inman U (1975) *Toward a Theory of Nursing Care.* Royal College of Nursing, London.

Lahiff M (1982) The Social Context of Nursing Research: a Sociological Analysis. Unpublished dissertation for Msc (Social Research), University of Surrey.

Lahiff M (1984) Attitudes to continuing education. *Nursing Times.* 80(2).

Lelean S and Clarke M (1990) Research resource development in the United Kingdom. *International Journal of Nursing Studies.* 27(2).

MacGuire J (1969) *Threshold to Nursing.* Bell, London.

MacGuire J (1970) The nurse/graduate in the United Kingdom: career paths. *International Nursing Review.* 18(4).

Manton J (1965) *Elizabeth Garrett Anderson.* Methuen, London.

McFarlane J K (1976) The Role of Research and the Development of Nursing Theory. *Journal of Advanced Nursing.* 1: 443–51.

McGann S (1992) *The Battle of the Nurses.* Scutari, London.

Menzies I. (1960) Functioning of social systems as a defence against anxiety. *Human Relations.* 13(2) May: 95–121. Subsequently republished as a Tavistock Monograph (1970).

Norton D (1985) A veteran's view of research in nursing. In Hawthorn P J (ed.) *Proceedings of the RCN Research Society Annual Conference.*

Nursing Times Editorial (1967) A research unit. *Nursing Times.* 63(49): 1637.

O'Meara S and Dickson R (1996) Use of nasogastric tubes for elective laparotomy. *Nursing Standard.* 10(41) 3 July.

Ouseley M H (1959) The case for a nursing research council. *Nursing Mirror.* 109(2840): xi–xii.

Owen G (1984) The Development of Degree Courses in Nursing Education – in Historical and Professional Context. Occasional Paper 4, Polytechnic of the South Bank, London.

Payne J (1983) Researchers 'Unpopular' nurses told. *Nursing Times.* 8 June: 20.

Reinkemeyer M H (1966) The Limited Impact of University Programmes in Nursing: A British Case Study. Unpublished PhD thesis, University of California.

Report of the Committee on Nursing (1972) (Chairman Asa Briggs) Cmnd 5115. HMSO, London.

Salvage J (1996) The games we play. Editorial, *Nursing Times* 92(19) 8 May.

Simpson H M (1971) 13th Nursing Mirror Lecture: Research, the first steps. *Nursing Mirror,* 12 March.
Stein L I (1968) The doctor/nurse game. *American Journal of Nursing* 68: 101–5.
Thompson A M C (ed.) (1968) *Bibliography of Nursing 1859–1960.* Royal College of Nursing, London.
Thompson A M C (ed.) (1974) *Bibliography of Nursing 1961–1970.* Royal College of Nursing, London.
Tierney A (1996) Nursing research at the University of Edinburgh. *Nursing Standard* 10(48) 21 August.
Walby S and Greenwell J, with Mackay L and Soothill K (1994) *Medicine and Nursing.* Sage, London.
Witz A (1992) *Professions and Patriarchy.* Routledge, London.

Further reading

Clay T (1987) *Nurses: Power and Politics.* Heinemann, London.
Davies C (ed.) (1980) A constant casualty: nurse education in Britain and the USA to 1939. In *Rewriting Nursing History.* Croom Helm, London.
Mackay L (1989) *Nursing a Problem.* Open University Press, Milton Keynes.
Salvage J (1985) *The Politics of Nursing.* Heinemann, London.
Soothill K, Mackay L and Webb C (eds) (1995) *Interprofessional Relations in Health Care.* Edward Arnold, London.
White R (ed.) (1988) *Political Issues in Nursing: Past, Present and Future.* John Wiley, Chichester.
Wieczorek R R (ed.) (1984) *Power, Politics, and Policy in Nursing.* Springer, New York.

4

Where do ideas come from?
Setting research agendas

Maria Lorentzon

This chapter focuses on nursing research and its management in Britain. The background to commissioning health services research within the Department of Health is outlined, together with the main milestones in NHS research from the 1970s to the present. Committee membership is examined and funding policies and sources are assessed. A literature search of the popular British nursing journals from 1992–94 was undertaken to explore various aspects of research management. Comparative material is drawn from the North American nursing journals. The chapter reviews and responds to the challenges of government directives, such as the NHS Research and Development Strategy, the Nursing Strategy for Nursing, Midwifery and Health Visiting, the findings of the Taskforce, the Research Assessment Exercise and the Culyer initiative. Emphasis is placed on strengthened collaboration between managers, educationalists, researchers and clinicians both within and outside nursing, midwifery and health visiting and an evaluation is given of the nurses' role in multidisciplinary research.

Introduction

Ideas and their origin have occupied the thoughts of philosophers over many centuries. While idealists have stressed intrinsic human values as the foundation for a civilized society shaped by the Judeo-Christian and earlier classical tradition, materialist philosophers, for instance Karl Marx, emphasize that ideas are generated from and sustained by material conditions. It could be argued that nursing in Britain can be seen as fitting into several broad phases: the pre-Protestant Reformation period, when most of the available medical, nursing and social care was provided within religious orders; the period from the sixteenth century following the closure of the monasteries by Henry VIII which also included the destruction of the monastic health care ethos, with the gin-sodden Dickensian Sairy Gamp as the prototype nurse; and the nineteenth century reform period dominated by Nightingale and the modern, professionalizing period (Lorentzon, 1992). A mix of idealism and pragmatism gave the Nightingale reform its peculiar potency. However, it is important to remember that Nightingale tempered her vocational approach to nursing with evidence based on systematic observation (Nightingale, 1859). In linking ideals viewed as 'natural in women' with devotion to hard work and self-abnegation a tradition was born (or resurrected), which provided maximum value for the health service.

Various models of professionalisation exist in sociological literature and it is not possible to deal with them all fully in this introductory section. There is a common thread running through most of these: the stress on autonomy and control over knowledge and the right to practise (Freidson, 1975). Nursing can be seen as having less control over its knowledge base than medicine. In this context it is important to remember that medicine has established itself as a profession over hundreds of years and has acquired a high level of legitimacy and prestige. It is, however, important to acknowledge that doctors from different specialisms perceive themselves as having different degrees of power. General practice has traditionally been viewed as a less prestigious branch of medicine than, say, cardiac surgery. Recent government reforms have, however, resulted in partial reorientation of these relationships with their increasing emphasis on a primary care-led NHS. This change in policy has affected both general practitioners and other primary care health workers and has resulted in the increasing prominence of primary care-based research.

Development of a credible research base in nursing, with ideas distinct from, but often complementary to, those propagated by other health professionals, has been part of this knowledge-based professionalization, providing a contrast with the earlier vocational approach. Emphasis on class and gender issues as influential on the evaluation of ideas in nursing has opened the door to critical interpretations of the power-base which nursing occupies in comparison to, say, medicine. The propagation of ideas which do not necessarily mirror medical priorities has been part of this intellectual emancipation and some of the milestones in this process within the British health service will be described below. The full impact of this important process cannot be adequately dealt with in this introduction but is clearly related to the capacity of nurses to generate research ideas. A gradual movement from subordination to partnerships between nurses in clinical, education and research roles and more powerful health professionals is taking place, albeit at a comparatively slow pace. In this context it is essential to distinguish between reality and pure ideology.

Gender issues are important in nursing which has a majority of women in its workforce. Feminism is relevant in this context. Power relationships between women and men in nursing are complex and no simple conclusions can be drawn about the influence of feminist thought on the profession. Because of this complexity it is difficult to assess the current impact of feminism on the nursing research agenda, although there has been some interesting debate in this area (Webb, 1984, 1993; Savage, 1987).

Formal networks to facilitate the careers of women in senior NHS management have also been established, such as the NHS Women's Unit set up in the early 1990s as a result of the government sponsored Opportunity 2000. Such structures benefit executive nurses as well as other female managers and are likely to influence the agenda for management, which in turn shapes clinical practice, education and research.

Influence by nurses as individuals and by nursing as a collective entity is exercised in a number of ways. Many of these may be viewed as the evolution of parallel structures to those set up by more powerful professionals, for example doctors. Nightingale created systems for 'separate' development, which ensured that while following doctors' orders about the *medical* treatment of patients, nurses were not directly managed by doctors. Cynics may observe that the drift of academic nurses into comparatively non-medicalized areas, such as care of the elderly, is more an avoidance of medical power and a craving for nurse autonomy than genuine preference for the specialty itself. The same argument may be advanced in seeking to explain the current intensified interest shown by nurses in qualitative social science research, leaving quantitative, 'hard' biomedical research to medical colleagues. Whether these explanations are partially true or not, there can be no doubt that complex power relations underlie the setting of a research agenda for nursing in the late 1990s which will therefore be unlikely to truly mirror the real needs of the service without contamination by pragmatism based on 'the art of the possible'. These power dynamics in the NHS context can be seen in the Culyer Report (DoH, 1994a) which will be discussed later. Although the report is called 'Supporting Research and Development in the NHS', there is no direct mention of nursing research in this paper, which relates to future funding of R&D in the health service. The availability of research grants to academic departments of nursing is minimal compared to medicine, based on personal observation by the author and other evidence, for instance the poor performance of departments of nursing in the 1992 University Research Assessment Exercise (RAE), which will be discussed later. The more recent 1996 RAE will be briefly reviewed. The degree of success with which different health professions manage to determine their own research agendas and to attract funding in order to achieve their stated objectives is largely conditional on overall influence within the health service and in society at large.

Commissioning research by the Department of Health: an overview

A search of the relevant literature reveals that policy-making in the area of research commissioning by government is not new. The method whereby government funds are distributed for research in the health service is clearly important for the various groups involved, for example, nurses. This will, to a great extent, influence research agendas, such as those underlying the commissioning of research by the government.

The main principles of research commissioning by the Department of Health are set out in a report by the Central Policy Review Staff under the direction of Lord Rothschild on the *Organisation and Management of Government Research and Development (Cmnd 4814)* (1971) as referred to by Lorentzon (1993). Recommendations arising from this report were accepted in a White Paper, *Framework for Government Research and Development (Cmnd 5046)* (1972) and included three main policy developments. These are described by Kogan, Korman and Henkel (1980) as follows:

1 The introduction of the customer–contractor relationship which would require the DHSS to specify needs as customers which researchers, as contractors, would then implement;
2 the appointment of an advisory Chief Scientist and an executive Director of Research and Development;
3 the transfer of research funds from three of the five research councils to government departments with the closest interest in their field of research. This was intended to enable . . . the DHSS to commission work through the Medical Research Councils (MRC). (pp. 1–2)

Research Liaison Groups were set up at the Department of Health and Social Security to propagate communication between policy makers and scientific advisors.

Following the Griffiths-inspired NHS management reorganization, R&D activities in the health service were re-evaluated and a number of shortcomings identified. These were set out in a Report by the Nuffield Provincial Hospitals Trust (1985). A less bureaucratic approach to commissioning government research was recommended. There was also strong emphasis on the need to ensure that research findings were implemented. It was observed that: 'any review of health services research and its place in medical care particularly points to . . . the failure to develop and maintain multidisciplinary research teams' (p. 9). Reference to poor research collaboration between members of different disciplines is significant and differential access to funding and influence in setting research agendas are clearly pertinent factors in this context, as discussed above. Significant reference to medical care is made in this criticism about the poor coordination of the multidisciplinary research team.

Following NHS reforms arising from recommendations in the White Papers *Working for Patients* (1989a) and *Caring for People* (1989b) a report entitled *Research for Health* (1991) was published by the Research and Development Division of the Department of Health. The report focused on research and development needs in the NHS set in the context of policy interests within the Department of Health. A common focus would be established in its Research and Development Division of the Department of Health. The responsibility for appointing Directors of Research and Development was given to the 14 Regional Health Authorities. (The subsequent reduction of RHAs and their abolition in April 1996 and the increasing power of the health market have had an impact on this strategy.) A Central Research and Development Committee was established to direct R&D within the NHS and it included two nurse members. The key points in *Research for Health* (1991) can be summarized as follows:

1   Research and development is an essential activity in which there must be sufficient investment to establish a coherent programme.
2   Responsibility for the programme will rest largely with the regions who develop, implement and are accountable for regional R&D programmes within a national framework.
3   Regional R&D programmes will be resourced from regional funds; in addition regions will have contracts with the centre to manage R&D in a number of priority areas of national importance which will be funded centrally.
4   Development of the programme will depend on close collaboration between universities and the NHS and these links will need to be reflected in regional arrangements.
5   The programme presents the opportunity of working towards a coherent national programme with the MRC, the Charities and industry. (p. 4)

The revised 1993(a) edition of *Research for Health* outlines in some detail the collaborative networks between the Department of Health and other bodies, which promote and fund R&D in the health service in relation to specific priority areas (see below). A new concordat between the Government Health Departments and the Medical Research Council was negotiated in 1991. It was noted that:

> The main emphasis of MRC-supported work is on biomedical research, while the focus of the health departments is on applied health research, including health services research and operational research. There is a common interest in public health and in clinical trials. (p. 5)

Recent stress on evidence-based health care has centred on randomized controlled trials. This provides a focus for debate about the impact of data arising from such studies on the nation's health.

The role of the Economic and Social Research Council in supporting health service research is emphasized and:

> in 1993 the Department of Health and the Economic and Social Research Council agreed a strategic alliance to mark closer working between the two agencies on health and social services research. (p. 5)

Nursing interests are not likely to figure prominently on Department of Health or NHS research agendas with such marked medical dominance in leadership positions unless powerful informal networks exist to ensure that priorities identified by nurses figure on the national R&D programmes for health service research. With this in mind it is encouraging to note that priorities for research and development in the NHS are broad, including areas within the following 'perspectives':

- disease-related
- management and organization
- client groups
- consumers
- health technologies
- methodologies.

Special Research Liaison Committees (RLC) have been established to bring together funding bodies in the public and private sectors. One such group, the Cardiovascular and Stroke RLC includes the MRC, British Heart Foundation, Wellcome Trust, Stroke Association and the Department of Health. It might be assumed that the membership of these organizations will strongly influence the resulting research agendas. For instance, the patient perspective will be represented by the Stroke Association and all health professions would, potentially, find a voice through the Department of Health. This should ensure that nursing interests are part of the agenda, as discussed below.

The Health Technology Forum focuses on coordinating new and existing technologies and health care interventions, which are relevant to the NHS. Research collaboration with industry has increased in recent years and the Department of Health is also working closely with the Office of Science and Technology (OST, 1993). The White Paper *Realising our Potential* (OST, 1993) recognizes the contribution of science and technology to public health and quality of life. It promotes a wider awareness of the value to the NHS which can be derived from research, for example in the field of pharmaceuticals.

Another forum for cross-national research is the Cochrane Centre, which is actively promoting international collaboration in the area of randomized controlled trials (RCTs) within health care. The Centre contributes the first element of the information systems strategy supporting the R&D programme and was opened in 1992. It is directed by Ian Chalmers and has been set up to assist specialists in a wide range of fields to prepare, maintain and disseminate systematic reviews of randomized controlled trials of health care. This information is essential in order to make well-informed decisions about health care and related research.

The NHS Centre for Reviews and Dissemination has also been set up at York University to undertake sytematic reviews of research findings. The remit of the centre includes a variety of research approaches other than controlled trials and the delivery and organization of health care as well as effective treatments.

A recurring theme throughout this book is that systematic reviews and their dissemination are regarded as central to a market-orientated health service in order to promote the use of 'tried and tested' health care. Getting Research into Purchasing and Practice (GRiPP) is one such initiative designed to inform clinicians and purchasers about the effectiveness or otherwise of a range of treatments based on the evidence of clinical trials (Dunning, McQuay and Milne, 1994). Four clinical areas were considered. These were: the use of grommet surgery for children; dilation and currettage (D and C); the use of cortico-steroids in pre-term delivery; and the management of stroke services. All four areas are very much orientated to medical practice but systematic reviews of nursing interventions have since been initiated. In 1993, Nicky Cullum, a nurse, working at that time with Karen Luker, one of the two nurse members of the DoH R&D committee (see below) was commissioned to undertake a critical review of the community nursing management of leg ulcers (Cullum, 1994). Her review showed that a number of RCTs demonstrated the effectiveness of some treatments but further studies were required to provide more conclusive evidence.

Thus the 1990s have witnessed increasing 'evidence' through a network of centres and databases. Databases established in this manner are thought to encompass research-based information that is valid and reliable, which in turn is used for drafting clinical guidelines and protocols. French (1996) describes how a consortium of educators and health care providers worked collaboratively to train and provide link practitioners to take evidence-based practice forward, including 'the development of consensus guidelines for best practice'.

While there can be no doubt that the emphasis on evidence-based health care, whether it be in nursing or medicine, provides an answer to those who bemoan the lack of use made of research findings, some caution is needed. Nurses must beware of uncritically adopting an approach specifically developed for medicine and heavily orientated to RCTs. Since much nursing research has not been generated by means of an RCT, the fundamental question remains, 'What is evidence in nursing?' A general answer which is likely to meet near-universal approval might be that evidence is any data which contribute to improved patient care. This is, however, such a wide-open response as to make it almost meaningless.

Inclusion of only RCT data, however, is too restricting not only in nursing but also in medicine and other health disciplines. This point is especially relevant when addressing issues related to complex areas such as palliative care in which the randomization of dying people into groups for intervention and non-intervention presents ethical dilemmas. All health professionals must unite their efforts to grapple with these issues and be prepared to let go of old certainties, crossing both professional and research boundaries in the process.

Membership of committees is clearly important in setting research agendas. It is significant that whereas total membership of the Central Research and Development Committee is 32, it includes 16 doctors and only three nurses. Among the Regional Directors of Research and Development appointed before the merger of RHAs in 1993, 11 out of 13 were doctors (North-West Thames had not made an appointment when North-East and North-West Thames Regions were merged). This prominence of doctors on decision-making bodies is likely to have an impact on the success or otherwise of proposed plans for nursing research in the NHS.

While no overt medical dominance is evident in the topic areas listed above, it is important for nurses and other health professionals to be vigilant in ensuring that the R&D agenda for the health service remains balanced including priorities of all clinicians intent on providing an adequate and flexible service for clients.

Formulating a strategy for nursing research and development

The need for a strategic approach to nursing research and development in the United Kingdom was gradually acknowledged following publication of an overall Strategy for Nursing in 1989 (1989c). The original intention was to weave in research themes under all main headings (practice, education and management) thereby obviating the need for a separate research strategy and conveying an integrated approach between research on the one hand and specialist areas of nursing practice on the other. Integration between nursing practice, education and research fits in with an holistic approach to health care. Clinical practice is thus thought to be directly influenced by education and research developments. This original view, however, was revised in the light of experience and Dame Anne Poole, then Chief Nursing Officer at the Department of Health, began a discussion about the main points for inclusion in the new Research Strategy in the early 1990s. A number of nurses in key positions and other experts were consulted, including members of the group of regional representatives on nursing research, of which the author was a member at that time. This membership was intended to represent clinical, academic and management interests related to nursing research. A three-day workshop was organized in 1991 at Wonersh, Surrey, to crystallize the main issues.

Following the retirement of Dame Anne and the appointment of Yvonne Moores as Chief Nursing Officer, a taskforce was established in 1992, chaired by Professor Adrian Webb (then at Loughborough, now at Glamorgan University) to complete the strategy. It is interesting to note that three out of only seven taskforce members were non-nurses. Membership of the group of which almost 50 per cent were non-nurses is an interesting factor in determining nursing influence on its own research agenda. In contrast the group which prepared the 1994 therapists' position statement (DoH, 1994b), which will be discussed later, consisted entirely of members of those professions. The taskforce reported in 1993 and the strategy was launched at a conference staged at Lancaster Hotel, London, in 1994. Emphasis in the programme was on multidisciplinary research, and R&D priorities in nursing as well as in therapy professions were addressed. Two out of three panel discussions were chaired by professors of medicine. The main report was published by the Department of Health and the Annexes by the Royal College of Nursing. It is important to note that Christine Hancock, General Secretary of the RCN, was a former member of the Briggs Committee (1972), which produced an important report stressing the need for nursing to become more research-based.

Recommendations arising out of the Taskforce Report are wide-ranging, focusing on:

- structure and organisation
- research, education and training
- funding for research
- integrating research and development.

It would seem that the second and third priority areas are the most essential in order to begin the generation of research ideas and to initiate projects. Without sound research education nurses are unlikely to be in a position to distinguish between viable and trivial ideas for research. The value of such education cannot be over-emphasized in the climate of research competition prevailing in today's health service and related academic departments. Without funding, research cannot be commenced, however worthy the underlying ideas may be. The combined impact of economic recession and government monetarist policies since 1979 has made the likelihood of funding for 'blue sky' research harder to obtain. In its broadest sense, 'blue sky' research refers to longer-term research which permits the pursuit of innovative ideas rather than responsive research which is set by external agendas. Fells, Professor of Energy Conversion, at Newcastle University, writes: 'Creative scientific research is being stifled by a materialistic society, marketplace economics and the dominating influence of industrialists on the research councils' (Fells, 1996). 'Politicians,' Fells suggests, 'know nothing of the fragile process of creativity and bow to the influence of businessmen and industrialists who talk persuasively of the "bottom-line".' Nurse researchers find themselves similarly constrained. Blue sky research still has an important role to play as a means of maintaining creativity and providing a pool of ideas from which to set longer-term agendas as well as responding to the more immediate needs determined by the NHS Research and Development Division.

Furthermore, the Nursing Research Strategy recommends that the Department of Health undertake an internal appraisal to ensure that:

- there is a coherent and high profile approach to research in nursing, midwifery and health visiting
- the nursing dimension is fully recognized and funded wherever it is relevant to a commissioned programme or project

- a nursing research dimension – especially relating to the evaluation of current and innovative practices and procedures – be firmly embedded in the refocused resources, which the Department devotes to research units, with each appropriate unit containing an identifiable element of nursing research.

The importance of research training is stressed and the recommendation is made that the Director of Research and Development at the Department of Health should:

initiate discussions with the Office of Science and Technology (OST) and the Research Councils to obtain additional funds for an expanded programme of research training of health services staff and for the nursing profession, in particular. An enhanced programme of research training should be a key feature of the concordant between the Medical Research Council (MRC) and the Department of Health (DoH) and of the agreement being established with the Economic and Social Research Council (ESRC). (p. 13)

Assessment of education and research in university departments of nursing

Having achieved publication and launch of this strategy which includes many practical recommendations for forthcoming nursing research, where would this lead? How likely are nurses to attract necessary research funds in a competitive market in view of the poor performance by university departments of nursing in the 1992 Research Assessment Exercise? (The Research Assessment Exercise is a means adopted by the Higher Education Funding Council for England for measuring research performance of university departments, using a scale from 5+, indicating international research excellence in most areas, to 1, which denotes total lack of research activity. The rating is based on three main factors: research funding, publication record by academic staff and number of research students being supervised.) Tierney (1994) observed that nursing was rated lowest of all 72 subjects reviewed in 1992. Out of 29 academic nursing departments assessed, 17 received the lowest possible rating and only five were awarded an average or above average rating. The comparative youth of many departments and the orientation towards professional education rather than research may be factors explaining this poor research performance. However, it is clearly a matter for concern and is unlikely to be helpful in attracting research funds unless these departments demonstrate radical improvement in the 1996 exercise. First impressions suggest they have not. However, a number of established departments did rather better, with the University of London's King's College achieving the much sought-after '5' rating.

Some departments decided to improve their chances by being assessed alongside colleagues from departments such as education and social policy.

But in considering the generally low ratings of nursing departments in the recent University Research Assessment Exercise it is interesting to speculate about the best strategy for improving the likely scores in the year 2000. Most departments of nursing still concentrate mainly on professional education and research activity is minimal. Proposals have been made to concentrate university research in a few élite institutions, which is unlikely to favour nursing. But thought is already being given as to how to change this. University departments of nursing are already beginning to plan their research strategies to improve their research output for the millennium. The result of the 1996 assessment provides some evidence of the current strength of the British nursing research base. There can be no doubt that it is strengthening. The *Journal of Advanced Nursing,* a British journal, was rated fifth from the top of the international Social Science Citation Index nursing section in 1994, based on the number of times its articles were referred to in publications by other authors.

The future of research in nursing will clearly be influenced by the current reorganization of nurse education. The shift from the NHS to the higher education sector places student nurses within a research-oriented environment. Although the currently poor research performance by nursing departments may be partly caused by the emphasis on nurse education rather than on research, this is likely to change gradually as these departments mature and more staff attain their doctoral degrees.

Nursing research, however, will need to be set firmly within the competitive environment prevailing in the British health service and academic environments. In *A Vision for the Future – The Nursing, Midwifery and Health Visiting Contribution to Health and Health Care* (NHSME, 1993) the NHS Management Executive outlines priorities for the future. Emphasis is placed on working in partnership with all health professionals, patients and their carers. Five ways of achieving this are suggested:

- quality/outcome assessment and audit
- accountability for practice
- clinical and professional leadership, clinical research and supervision
- purchasing and commissioning
- education and personal development.

It is rather bizarre to note that clinical research is linked with 'supervision' rather than with 'education and personal development'. Linkage of clinical research with supervision appears to denote a managerial approach to research in nursing. While it is clearly important to ensure that competent practitioners are informed by up-to-date research findings and that managers exercise supervision to enable this learning process, clinical research is surely more directly associated with education and personal development. It is also disappointing to observe that the target, following reference to clinical research, simply relates to the development of clinical and professional leadership as part of a corporate management agenda, again emphasizing management rather than academic research aims. There would seem to be evidence that lip service is still paid to nursing research in the NHS without genuine intent to focus specifically on research priorities with the allocation of the necessary resources.

Mention has been made in Chapter 3 of professionalization theories and in this chapter, although further study would still be needed by the keen reader to cover all the relevant literature. However, there can be no doubt that the common thread running through most concepts of what a profession is relates to *control over knowledge and practice* and thus to *the level of autonomy* exercised by a particular occupational group.

The development of a solid position for nursing within academia is therefore important. It could thus be argued that the professionalization of nursing in recent years has taken place partly through the relocation of nurse education from the NHS to universities with the creation of numerous Chairs and other senior academic posts. It is clearly imperative for nurses in these posts to justify their position through the demonstration of credible research achievements based on new and creative ideas. Unless such evidence of research activity is forthcoming with prominent input to the health service research agenda, nursing is likely to be abandoned to sit on the sidelines, while established professionals and academics move in to take the prizes.

Multidisciplinary research collaboration in the NHS – fact or fiction?

An ideological commitment to multidisciplinary work within a variety of areas in the NHS has prevailed for the last few decades and has intensified in recent years. Less powerful groups, such as nurses, have seized this opportunity to further their aims in clinical practice, education, management and research which could not be adequately promoted in a unidisciplinary nursing setting. Multidisciplinary approaches have been supported most forcefully by less influential groups: medical enthusiasm in this respect would appear lukewarm and anecdotal evidence points to a lack of interest in multidisciplinary education by medical students in some medical schools.

Questions need to be asked about the real benefits of multidisciplinary collaboration in the health service and the extent to which the approach is truly implemented. There must be clear guidelines related to areas of work, which specifically lend themselves to this approach and others where a unidisciplinary style would appear more appropriate. There is a need to develop clear criteria for multidisciplinary work at both generalist and specialist levels. This applies not only to collaboration between discrete professional groups, but to subgroups within generic professions such as medicine and nursing. Multidisciplinary collaboration in more broadly based health and social care fields, such as the care of elderly people, is, however, ideal in drawing on the skills of all disciplines involved. For example, a recent study was undertaken to evaluate the integration of health and social care for elderly people in one local authority. The research was commissioned by a primary health care chief executive in conjunction with social workers. Members of the primary health care team participated with the research team which included two nurses, a sociologist and an economist (Smith *et al.* 1996).

Variable levels of power and influence in academic and health service settings will clearly influence partnerships formed to conduct multidisciplinary research and this could lead to competition and sometimes to conflict. Should precious energy be wasted in power struggles, which could more profitably be devoted to the promotion of effective health care for patients? This question needs to be addressed when examining recommendations in various Department of Health reports, which tend to support multidisciplinarity in R&D. Patient needs must remain the chief focus. This is reflected in the Nursing Research Initiative for Scotland led by Jenny Hunt, which emphasizes patient focus and multidisciplinary research. While professionalization issues are important for nurses, service aspects are clearly at the centre of the debate (NRIS, 1996). The division of health service labour must also be viewed in this light. It is, however, important for nurses to beware of accepting medical tasks uncritically, as previously discussed. A similar argument can be made about multidisciplinary research. If the nurse's role is simply that of routine data collector in medically led projects, warning bells must be sounded. Equal partnerships in service, education and research must be the aim.

The 1993(a) edition of *Research for Health* refers to support for the creation of a number of multidisciplinary centres for research and development. Specific reference was made to the establishment of a 'new centre for Research and Development in Primary Health Care'. The aim would be to 'build up a multidisciplinary group, transcending traditional disciplinary boundaries in order to create a stimulating environment for health services research' (p. 28). It would appear that primary care is viewed as an ideal seed-bed to generate multidisciplinary research for reasons discussed above.

It is interesting to note the emphasis on 'applied' and 'operational' R&D as requiring a 'wide range of research skills . . . coming from a variety of backgrounds and disciplines' (p. 28). Primary health care and public health seem to be the most obvious areas of multidisciplinary work where egalitarian collaboration would have some hope of success. Questions, however, must be asked about the extent to which true multidisciplinary research collaboration can be extensively fostered in biomedical settings. While there is some evidence that nurses are rising from their subservient role of pure data collectors, for example in cancer research, it will be interesting to compare the progress of multidisciplinary research in specialist/fundamental and generalist/applied areas in the health service and related academic departments. It is significant that the *Report of the Taskforce on the Strategy for Research in Nursing, Midwifery and Health Visiting* (DoH, 1993b) recommended the creation of centres for research-led practice and that the Department of Health responded by allocating funding for 'a new multidisciplinary centre for research-led practice' (p. 27). While there could be many reasons why a multidisciplinary approach would enrich research in the nursing professions, it should not be a taken-for-granted notion. Was there ever an option to establish a separate centre devoted specifically to the many possible research topics, which could be identified in the numerous nursing specialities developing in the UK? Were nurses forced to accept multidisciplinarity as the only choice on offer? Committee membership at the Department of Health and within regions has already been discussed. Comparatively low numbers of nurse members on all decision-making bodies could lay them open to the charge of not fully representing nursing needs and priorities for R&D in spite of the contention that the Central R&D Committee (CRDC) draws on the 'collective expertise of its multidisciplinary membership' in achieving 'consistency of approach' (p. 9).

It is interesting to note that the taken-for-granted notion that a multi-disciplinary approach to R&D is necessarily beneficial for nurses was challenged in various presentations and panel discussions during the 1994 Conference to launch the Taskforce Report and in a later editorial by this author (Lorentzon, 1995). It is therefore important to study the recommendations of the taskforce in some detail.

While the assumption that a multidisciplinary base is the ideal setting for nursing research is clearly made in *Research for Health* (1991, 1993a) this is by no means the case in the *Report of the Taskforce on the Strategy for Research in Nursing, Midwifery and Health Visiting* (1993b). There are few direct references to multidisciplinary R&D and more stress on the need to provide additional resources for nursing research to allow the 'catching up' process with other professions to take place in the areas of research training, funding and general expansion. The ambivalence between strong awareness that such resources are needed and the fear that 'separate development' may isolate nursing research is apparent throughout the Report. While some support was given to establishment of a separate Research Council for Nursing there was also acknowledgement that 'research in nursing and the nursing professions is not a special case; it is but an important part of a larger whole' (p. 7). Taking the latter view to its furthest extreme, one conclusion which might be drawn is that research in nursing should be wholly encompassed within a body of health services research. This suggestion is rejected, however, and attention is drawn to valuable work conducted within academic nursing departments. The aim should be to create 'a cadre of nurse researchers capable of contributing to health care research generally as well as to research in nursing' (p. 9) This could be 'set alongside the illustrious tradition of basic clinical biomedical research' (p. 8). Reading the Taskforce Report, one theme emerges clearly: the need to balance separate nursing research needs and priorities with the overall aims and objectives of health services research. While *Research for Health* conveys a strong link between nursing and multidisciplinary R&D to the point of blurring and almost obliterating the boundaries between them, this is not the case in the Taskforce Report as highlighted above.

Having explored support for multidisciplinary research in *Research for Health* and the *Report of the Taskforce on the Strategy for Research in Nursing, Midwifery and Health Visiting* similar themes will be examined in *Research and Development in Occupational Therapy, Physiotherapy and Speech and Language Therapy: a Position Statement* (1994b) and *Supporting Research and Development in the NHS* (Culyer Report 1994a). The latter report relates to new arrangements for funding R&D in the NHS. The exact terms of reference for the committee, chaired by Professor Anthony Culyer of the University of York, were: 'to consider whether to recommend changes in the conduct and support of Research' and 'Development (R&D) in and by the NHS, and if so to advise on alternative funding and support mechanisms for R&D, including transitional measures within available resources' (p. 7).

In comparing memberships of the taskforce set up to consider nursing research and the therapy professions group convened to draft the position statement, it is significant that the former consisted of only four members representing the nursing professions out of a total membership of seven, whereas all 13 members of the therapy professions group belonged to those disciplines. Five out of ten members of the main Culyer Committee were doctors and three were general managers. No members represented nursing or therapy professions specifically, although Professor Tony Butterworth of Manchester University Department of Nursing was a member of a 'support group'. The Chairman was a Professor of Economics. This may have been intended to ensure impartiality in not assigning a health professional or manager to that role.

The position statement by therapists appeared more positive than the Taskforce Report on *A Strategy for Nursing Research* in relation to the subject of multidisciplinary work. This may partly reflect the small numbers in therapy professions and the consequent need to form alliances. There was positive encouragement to 'recognise the contribution that the therapy professions can and should be making to the multidisciplinary programme of health services research' (p. 1). Making reference to the Nursing Taskforce Report, emphasis was placed on the need to ensure that therapists are not disadvantaged in seeking 'mainstream research funding'. Stress was placed on the need to develop 'collaborative multidisciplinary research' (p. 4). Therapists should 'liaise with the Research and Development Directors on multidisciplinary initiatives' (p. 5). An appropriate balance between unidisciplinary and multidisciplinary research should be the aim

(p. 7). Active encouragement was given for academic therapy departments to be actively involved 'in the tendering process for multidisciplinary health care research programmes, being established by the Department of Health, NHS and the Research Councils' (p. 10).

The Culyer Report (1994a) focused on the need to 'recommend changes in the conduct and support of Research and Development (R&D) in and by the NHS' (p. 7). Recommendation was made to 'recast' the CRDC membership to 'ensure that the perspectives of NHS purchasers and providers and key commissioners of R&D, such as higher education institutions, research councils, charities and industry are adequately represented on the Committee' (p. 8). Reference was made to the need to provide funds to cover 'the direct costs of R&D' to 'professionals working in primary and community health care settings'. A recommendation was made for the creation of 'R&D commissioning units, accountable to the Director of Research and Development through the NHS Executive's Regional Offices' (p. 11). Although it is assumed that such units would have adequate representation from all health professions this is not clearly spelt out, nor is there any direct reference to multidisciplinary research.

Multidisciplinary collaboration in national and local R&D programmes are in line with current rhetoric. The reality means different things to the various players: it may represent a threat to more vulnerable groups with comparatively insecure status in the academic and professional hierarchy, but may, at the same time, ensure some part in the action where otherwise there would be no involvement by the less dominant groups. The most important issue, however, must be whether a multidisciplinary approach to health services research (HSR) benefits services for patients. Systematic comparative evaluation of research in similar areas, conducted within multidisciplinary and unidisciplinary teams and academic departments, should be conducted to demonstrate the respective benefits of both approaches. Based on the author's experience, overall benefit to the service must be the primary concern rather than narrow professional interests in securing research funding and prestige.

Managing nursing research in the 1990s: exploring the nursing press

Research by professionals in the NHS must be seen in the context of the new health market, introduced following the reforms in 1990. Debate in the mid-1990s centres on the need to convince purchasers that a research component should be integral to services commissioned from providers such as hospital and community health care trusts. In order to achieve this, nursing must demonstrate the value of its research activity. Nurses are themselves confident of its merit. Thus Luker, Professor of Community Nursing at Liverpool University, (1992) asserts that: 'in recent years there has been a growing recognition of the scientific merit and high quality of much nursing research' (p. 1151).

As a member of the Department of Health Central Research and Development Committee, Luker is in a prime position to determine whether this view extends beyond the boundaries of nursing. The performance of academic nursing departments in the 1992 Research Assessment Exercise, which has been discussed above, would seem to cast some doubt on the general credibility of academic nursing research. The need to convince purchasers that research by nurses and related to nursing is worthy of their consideration is not in doubt for Benton, former Director of Quality and Community Relations at East London and City Health Authority and currently employed within the Northern Region. In a paper written by Benton and Avery (1993) they confidently express the belief that:

> replacement of ritual behaviour with research-based practice can release resources which, we hope, providers and purchasers are innovative and imaginative enough to use wisely in achieving benefits for the population. (p. 30)

From the provider side Burroughs (1993), who worked within the Whittington Hospital Trust in North London, is equally positive in asserting that:

> research is fundamental to professional practice and that nurses must know that their practice is based on sound theoretical principles which are supported by available research. (p. 46)

Now more than ever before, initiatives such as the Cochrane and York databases of systematic reviews and GRiPP, described earlier in this chapter, give clinicians the opportunity to access research findings to support their practice.

The national status of nursing research is clearly influenced by many factors, not least the views of the Chief Nursing Officer at the Department of Health. Although Yvonne Moores is described as having 'set up numerous research projects' by Carlisle in a 1993 interview, the priorities for the near future were seen to include: 'a new strategy for nursing, strengthening the role of nurses in purchasing health care, the changing role of the midwife and nurse education, including PREP' (Carlisle, 1993a, p. 19).

Further references to the NHS Management Executive's 12 targets 'to encourage nursing, midwifery and health visiting to achieve the government's health reforms' (p. 9) and to 'the new vision for nursing' (Carlisle, 1993b) set the 1993 national agenda with no direct reference to research.

Stress is placed on the role of nursing in promoting the current health reforms. Research, however, would tend to be critical and challenging regarding policy issues in general and the new health market among them. Moores makes reference to the shift from secondary to primary health care and to the changes proposed in the Tomlinson Report (1992) (Carlisle, 1993a, p. 19).

The enthusiasm for a Tomlinson-style reduction in secondary care facilities expressed by Moores was found to be misplaced in her 1994 endorsement of a predicted '50 000 cut in the 130 000 current NHS beds by the turn of the century' (Carlisle, 1994, p. 6). These figures, originally produced by the Welsh Planning Forum, have since been described as 'inflated' by the forum's executive director, Morton Warner.

While a healthy scepticism regarding Department of Health policies must be part of any researcher's armoury, the stated intent by Virginia Bottomley, former Secretary of State for Health, to encourage nurses and doctors in adopting 'an evaluative culture' cannot be dismissed lightly nor her belief that: 'the Department of Health Research & Development strategy will ensure that knowledge based patient care becomes a reality across the NHS' (News, 1993a, *Nursing Standard*, p. 10).

The real proof of Department of Health commitment to nursing research will be the positive response to recommendations made in the *Report of the Taskforce on the Strategy for Research in Nursing, Midwifery and Health Visiting*, already described. One such consequence is the establishment of the Centre for Policy in Nursing Research, which is based at the London School of Hygiene and Tropical Medicine, but is a joint initiative between the School and the Royal College of Nursing. Funding for the Centre has been provided by the Nuffield Provincial Hospitals Trust. The remit of the Centre is to assess the current level of research activity in nursing and from this basis to develop policies for nursing research in the future.

Comments about the Taskforce Report in the nursing press are relevant to this discussion. Headlines announcing the launch of and describing the conference to discuss the Taskforce Report provide a flavour of reactions to its content. *Nursing Standard* reporter David Allen (1993) entitled his item 'Nursing research falls short'. He then went on to say:

> poor quality nursing research and a lack of national direction are impeding the developing of knowledge-based practice according to the Department of Health's new Strategy for Research. But extra funding has been ruled out. (p. 6)

A News item in a later issue of the *Nursing Standard* (1993b) was equally negatively headlined with 'Conference to discuss report criticising Nursing Research'. The anonymous reporter announced that: 'fears that a government report that criticised the quality of nursing research will be left on the shelf have been dismissed by the Department of Health' (p. 12). The reporter continued by stating that:

> the report claimed the amount and range of nursing research fell well short of what is required ... poor quality nursing research and the lack of a national direction are impeding development of knowledge-based practice. (p. 12)

The *Nursing Times* News (1993a) reported rejection by the then Minister of Health, Dr Mawhinney, of the suggestion 'that more funding should be put into nursing research to bring it into line with the medical profession' (p. 7).

Medical leadership in furthering implementation of the report's recommendations was suggested in that:

A Steering Group, chaired by Richard Himsworth, Director of Research and Development at East Anglia RHA, will coordinate the implementation of the report's recommendations. (p. 7)

More effective input to the debate was provided in reports by Downey (1993) and members of the RCN Research Advisory Group. Downey noted the lack of opportunities for nurses to develop a research career. Funding was a problem, but the report did not recommend 'ring fencing' nursing research moneys as this would make it a special case and not an integral part of overall health care research. Downey interviewed Barbara Wade at the Royal College of Nursing who supported nursing research as part of the mainstream, saying that: 'nursing research could really benefit from a multidisciplinary input. I think we have been far too purist for far too long' (Downey, 1993, p. 18).

The cynic may replace 'purist' with 'protectionist' as there would seem to be good cause to fear that nursing research would fare relatively badly in open competition for research resources in the NHS. There would seem to be evidence of the continuing marginalization of nursing *and* therapy research in the NHS: Culyer (DoH, 1994a) made no direct reference to nursing in his report on research funding the NHS and only brief mention of research by therapists. Nor was any such mention made in the NHSE report *Research and Development in the New NHS: Functions and Responsibilities'* (1994) which was based on Culyer's report. Virginia Bottomley's Press Release (December 1994c) announcing the new funding mechanism for NHS Research and Development, based on levies payable by purchasers, made mention only of 'medical advance' which would improve patient services (DoH, 1994c). As this strategy is implemented it is essential for nurses in NHS Trusts with research and practice development remits to be proactive, in order to ensure that their research priorities are represented.

Members of the RCN Research Advisory Group (1993) considered the Taskforce Report carefully and concluded that: 'the thrust of this strategy is to put nursing research within the HSR mainstream. To do so also means that nursing will receive few concessions or privileges' (p. 22). Lack of funding for nursing research by the MRC and ESRC was defined as a special problem by Christine Hancock of the Royal College of Nursing (*Nursing Standard* News, 1993c).

Nursing clearly cannot both preserve a protected separate status and become an equal partner in the NHS research community. In my view there can be no other way of advancing nursing research than through meritocracy. A challenging note is added by Professor T. Stacey, a Professor of Medicine, speaking at the 1994 conference launching the Taskforce Report, urging nurses 'not to use doctors as (research) models' because the medical profession had 'split itself up' into specialties fragmenting the overall thrust of integrated medical research as reported by Friend (1994). It would appear from this statement that nurses are encouraged to emphasize generic rather than separatist elements of their discipline in order to achieve maximum research impact. Action arising from the Taskforce Report Recommendations, which include emphasis on research training, was crucial in the year preceding the 1996 University Research Assessment Exercise. Education-based and ENB-funded research is essential as nurse education gradually transfers from the NHS to the higher education sector (*Nursing Times* News, 1993b; Clifford, 1994). Paradoxically, it was this process which partly contributed to nursing receiving the lowest research rating of all 72 subjects assessed in the 1992 University Research Assessment Exercise as new departments concentrating entirely on professional education were entered into the evaluation as discussed above. Thus Smith (1994) notes that: 'nursing has the dubious distinction of being the lowest rated subject area in the 1992 Research Selectivity Exercise. On a scale of 1 to 5, nursing achieved an average weighted rating of 2.2' (p. 385).

It has been argued that it is mainly the inability of nurses to attract substantial research funding which contributes to this low rating and the lack or prominence given to financing nursing research, for instance in the Culyer report, would seem to bear this out.

The Professor of Nursing at Manchester, Tony Butterworth, 'denies claims that a review system used to evaluate nursing research is biased' (*Nursing Times* News, 1993c). Butterworth, whose department was among the few which received the highest rating achieved by any nursing department, was a member of the assessment panel. A spirited defence of nursing research was provided by Marsland (1993), a Professor of Sociology, who cast doubt on the impartiality of the assessment process so ardently defended by Butterworth. Marsland maintained that he had no doubt that: 'the nursing research panel was a good deal more rigorous than many other panels, particularly those in the arts and social sciences' (p. 45).

Whatever may be the cause of nursing's poor research performance, Couchman (1994) is convinced that: 'politically driven management priorities are squeezing nursing research into a position where it cannot develop the profession's knowledge base' (p. 18). It is significant that on being appointed to the post of NHS Chief Executive, Alan Langlands, in his 'Agenda for nurse leaders' (interviewed by Naish, 1994) made no mention of nursing research.

Ambivalence seems to characterize British nursing research in the troubled mid-1990s. This contrasts sharply with the confidence expressed in the US journal *Nursing Management* in which Smeltzer and Hinshaw (1993) maintain that:

> It is important that the philosophy and strategic plan for a department of nursing support research programs which will guide current clinical and administrative decisions as well as long-term policy initiatives. Research also

contributes to the maturing of the science of nursing through generating and testing knowledge. (p. 42)

Concluding reflections

Having examined a number of documents related to nursing research, are we in a better position to determine where underlying ideas come from? The origins of ideas may vary: they may spring from the public or from professionals involved in the service. The real significance lies in the degree to which ideas result in action. This will depend on the extent to which nurses can attract research funding through enthusing others about their ideas. Total lack of reference to funding for nursing research in the Culyer Report does not bode well for the future. Anecdotal evidence in 1996 pointed to nursing, midwifery and health visiting research taking a back seat in the Culyer assessments of the costs of health service research to the NHS. Much of the available information is confidential. It is perhaps significant that such data are often labelled 'commercial, in confidence' although they relate to a statutory service – the British National Health Service. Bearing in mind the likelihood that nursing priorities will be comparatively low on the Culyer agenda, should protected funds be ring-. fenced for nursing research or should nurses enter the meritocratic fray of open competition for funding within the multidisciplinary setting? Would it not be preferable to risk defeat than to dwell in 'protected isolation'? Nurses must face these questions as they learn to become more politically astute and confident in asserting their claim to a share of available research funds. Ideas alone will not 'conquer the world', they have to be resourced in order to result in research action. Nurses who are competing with more influential colleagues will be well aware of this fact. They will know the difference between mere ideology and realistic ideas for research which are likely to attract funding and result in genuine benefit for patients.

References

Allen D (1993) Nursing research falls short. *Nursing Standard* 7(35): 6.

Benton D and Avery G (1993) Quality, research and ritual in nursing. *Nursing Standard* 7(49): 29–30.

Briggs A (1972) *Report on the Committee on Nursing*. HMSO, London.

Burroughs J (1993) Research-based approach to nursing care. *Senior Nurse* 13(6): 46–7.

Carlisle D (1993a) Moore's Code. *Nursing Times* 89(14): 19.

Carlisle D (1993b) NHS sets targets to speed up health reforms. *Nursing Times* 89(18): 9.

Carlisle D (1994) CNO's bed reduction figures discredited by new report. *Nursing Times* 90(26): 6.

Clifford C (1994) Nursing gets debated. *Nursing Management (UK)* 1(2): 18.

Couchman W (1994) Nursing research gets debased. *Nursing Mangement (UK)* 1(2): 18.

Cullum N (1994) Leg ulcer treatments: a critical review (parts 1 and 2). *Nursing Standard* 9(1) 28 Sept.: 29–33, 9(2) 5 Oct.: 32–6.

Department of Health (1989a) *Working for Patients* (White Paper). DoH/HMSO, London.

Department of Health (1989b) *Caring for People* (White Paper). DoH/HMSO, London.

Department of Health (1989c) *A Strategy for Nursing.* DoH/HMSO, London.

Department of Health (1990) *NHS and Community Care Act.* HMSO, London.

Department of Health (1991) *Research for Health.* DoH/HMSO, London.

Department of Health (1993a) *Research for Health* (2nd edn.). DoH/HMSO, London.

Department of Health (1993b) *Report of the Taskforce on the Strategy for Research in Nursing, Midwifery and Health Visiting.* DoH/HMSO, London.

Department of Health (1994a) *Supporting Research and Development in the NHS (Culyer Report)* HMSO, London.

Department of Health (1994b) *Research and Development in Occupational Therapy, Physiotherapy and Speech and Language Therapy: a Position Statement.* DoH/HMSO, London.

Department of Health (1994c) *Press Release: Virginia Bottomley Announces Radical New Funding Mechanism for NHS Research and Development.* Richmond House, London.

Department of Health and Social Security (1971). *The Organisation and Management of Government Research and Development* (Rothschild Report, Cmnd. 4814). HMSO, London.

Department of Health and Social Security (1972). *Framework for Government Research and Development* (Cmnd. 5046). HMSO, London.

Downey R (1993) Inquiring minds. *Nursing Times* 89(22): 18.

Dunning M, McQuay H and Milne R (1994) Getting a GRiP. *Health Services Journal,* 104(5400), 28 April: 24–6.

Fells I (1996) Curiosity killed by bureaucrats. *Guardian,* 19 November.

Freidson E (1975) *Profession of Medicine.* Dodd, Mead, New York.

French B (1996) Networking for research dissemination: collaboration between education and practice. *NT research* 1(2): 113–18.

Friend B (1994) Academic says there is no such thing as nursing research. *Nursing Times* 90(20): 8.

Kogan M, Korman N and Henkel M (1980) *Government Commissioning of Research.* Department of Government, Brunel University.

Lorentzon M (1992) Medieval London: care of the sick. *Royal College of Nursing History of Nursing Society Journal* 4(2): 100–11.

Lorentzon M (1993) Research for health: managing the nursing input. *Journal of Nursing Management* 1: 39–46.

Lorentzon M (1995) Multidisciplinary collaboration: lifeline or drowning pool for nurse researchers? Guest Editorial. *Journal of Advanced Nursing* 22: 825–6.

Luker K (1992) Research and development in nursing: Guest Editorial. *Journal of Advanced Nursing* 17: 1151–2.

Marsland D (1993) Research and density. *Nursing Standard* 7(32): 45.

Naish J (1994) Langlands: Agenda for nurse leaders. *Nursing Management (UK)* 1(1): 6–8.

National Health Service Executive (1994) *Research and Development in the NEW NHS: Functions and Responsibilities.* HMSO, London.

National Health Service Management Executive (1993) *A Vision for the Future: The Nursing, Midwifery and Health Visiting Contribution to Health and Health Care.* HMSO, London.

News (1993a) *Nursing Standard* 7(42): 10.

News (1993b) *Nursing Standard* 8(9): 12.

News (1993c) *Nursing Standard* 8(11): 7.

News (1993a) *Nursing Times,* 89(20): 7.

News (1993b) *Nursing Times* 89(29): 6.

News (1993c) *Nursing Times* 89(2): 6.

Nightingale F (1859) (1980 reprint) *Notes on Nursing: What It Is and What It Is Not.* Churchill Livingstone, London.

Nuffield Provincial Hospitals Trust (1985) *A Fresh Look at Policies for Health Service Research and its Relevance to Management,* Occasional Paper 3. NPHT, London.

Nursing Research Initiative for Scotland (1996) *NRIS Newsletter,* 1 January.

Office of Science and Technology (1993) Realising our potential: a strategy for science, engineering and technology (White Paper). HMSO, London.

Royal College of Nursing Research Advisory Group (1993). Strategic thinking. *Nursing Standard* 7(38): 22.

Savage J (1987) *Nurses, Gender and Sexuality.* Heinemann Medical, London.

Smeltzer C M and Hinshaw A S (1993) Integrating research in a strategic plan. *Nursing Management (US)* 24(2): 42–4.

Smith L N (1994) An analysis and reflection on the quality of nursing research in 1992. *Journal of Advanced Nursing* 19: 385–93.

Smith P, Jennings J, Towers B and Mackintosh M (1996) The integration of health and social care for the elderly in one local authority. Unpublished Consultancy Report.

Tierney A (1994) An analysis of nursing's performance in the 1992 assessment of research in British universities. *Journal of Advanced Nursing* 19: 593–602.

Webb C (1984) Feminist methodology in nursing research. *Journal of Advanced Nursing* 9(3): 249–56.

Webb C (1993) Feminist research: definitions, methodology, methods and evaluation. *Journal of Advanced Nursing* 18(3): 416–23.

5

Discourse analysis: A tool for change in nursing policy, practice and research

Abigail Masterson

In this chapter, discourse analysis is proposed as a powerful tool to assist nurses to influence health care policies and research agendas and become politically astute. The author also demonstrates its huge potential for developing nursing and nursing practice. Discourse analysis takes up Wedderburn Tate's claim that 'documentation divorces the personal telling from the recording' and the need to put neglected groups of people on the health care and research agenda.

The author examines nursing's prevailing theoretical frameworks and highlights their limitations. The illuminatory and emancipatory powers of discourse analysis, especially when combined with critical theory, are emphasized. Nursing research studies using this combined approach are described. Finally the author considers some of the methodological issues associated with discourse analysis, including its tools and techniques; advantages and disadvantages; validity, reliability and rigour.

Introduction

In this chapter I define and describe discourse analysis in order to highlight its potential contribution to shaping nursing research agendas, policy and practice. Particular emphasis is given to the illuminatory and emancipatory powers of discourse analysis especially when combined with critical theory. To date there has been a lack of nursing research using this method although there is evidence to suggest that this situation is changing (Thompson, 1985; Elliot, 1989; Hiraki, 1992; Johnson, 1993; Masterson 1994).

The first half of the chapter draws on discourse analysis to present a case study of nursing and health policy. Nursing is the largest single occupation in the health services. Nurses are responsible for the majority of professional health care given in the UK, comprise more than half of all National Health Service (NHS) staff and consume nearly a quarter of all

expenditure on health. By comparison, the expenditure on nursing research is very small, accounting for only a tiny proportion of the total NHS R&D budget (DoH, 1992; Traynor and Rafferty, 1997). Health policy and the structures resulting from it, which shape and control nursing, are the outcome of governmental values and the negotiation and bargaining of powerful groups such as medicine and commerce in the health policy arena. Nurses have traditionally paid little attention to health policy, focusing instead on the micro level of care provision. Nursing, too, has tended to be ignored by policy-makers and policy analysts. In this chapter I aim to demonstrate how the techniques of discourse analysis can be used by nurses to shape and set their own agendas for policy, practice and research. In other words, discourse analysis will be promoted as a method with the potential to facilitate the exploration of nursing at a macro level.

I also examine the prevailing theoretical frameworks in nursing which emphasize holism and health and draw on critical theory to demonstrate the limitations of these approaches. Critical theorists contend that language plays a central role in reproducing power relations in society. Consequently discourses such as those contained in policy documents and professional publications identify the values that are important to a society and have a role in determining the structure of social institutions such as health services. However, while debates on health reform acknowledge values as being important, as yet there is little analysis of the values implicit in different models of health care and among different professional groups. Critical theory attempts to explain the social order in such a way that it itself becomes the catalyst which transforms this same social order.

In part 2 of the chapter I look at some of the methodological issues associated with discourse analysis. As a research method, discourse analysis, informed by critical theory, aims to reveal the mechanisms by which power is exercised. Drawing on the available literature in the field and using the construction of nursing within contemporary health policy as a case study, the need to put a critical theory perspective on nursing's research agenda will be advocated.

Part 1: Nursing and health policy: a case study

The original NHS discourse was based on a public service ethos committed to the treatment and (to a lesser extent) the prevention of disease. Universal coverage ensured care was provided free at the point of delivery from 'the cradle to the grave'. In recent years, the UK government, in common with all governments, is facing rising health costs, growing demand and the impact of demographic and technological change (Ham, 1992; Liss, 1993). There is some recognition by researchers and governments that people's health does not only depend on the amount and quality of health services, however well financed and managed. Nevertheless, while debates on health reform acknowledge values as being important, there is typically little analysis of the values implicit in some models of health care or of how values relate to people's health.

Health policy and the structures created by it are the result of governmental values, negotiation and bargaining (Ham, 1992). The creation of the NHS in 1948 resulting from the combined forces of the Labour movement, represented by the trade unions, the national coalition government's experience of central planning during the Second World War and Aneurin Bevan's leadership as the post-war Labour government's Minister of Health, is a case in point. Bevan negotiated a hard bargain (some commentators would say compromise) with the hospital consultants who were resistant to the idea of an NHS because they believed its creation would curb their clinical freedom and right to private practice. Bevan is said to have 'stuffed their mouths with gold' by agreeing to the option of private practice and access to pay beds in NHS hospitals for hospital consultants; a system of distinction awards with associated salary increases and a major role in the administration of the service at all levels.

As illustrated by the example of the hospital consultants and the Labour movement in the creation of the NHS, pressure groups attempt to influence policy-making and implementation at both national and local levels. Relationships between pressure groups and governments vary (for instance, the post-war Labour government had very different ideas and values about the NHS compared with the Conservative government of the mid-1980s). Ham (1992) uses Beer's (1969) work to suggest that it is producer groups, such as the British Medical Association (including the hospital consultants of the late 1940s) which have the greatest influence over policy formulation, implementation and outcome.

Nursing as the largest single occupation in health care is the largest producer group (Buchan, 1991). Nurses, it is often said, should therefore be a powerful group in the policy-making and implementation process, both because of their numbers and their ability to command public sympathy. As a producer group they are responsible for the majority of professional health care given in the UK, comprise more than half of all NHS staff and consume nearly a quarter of all health service expenditure (Beardshaw, 1992). Nursing is not homogenous, however, being composed of practitioners, educators, researchers and managers and being frequently divided into subgroups by speciality and place of work such as hospital or community, state or independent sector. This lack of homogeneity leads to fragmentation and a lack of consensus about the content and organization of nursing among groups as diverse as intensive care nurses and health visitors; community psychiatric nurses and orthopaedic nurses; or nursing lecturers and acute trust managers.

Traditionally nurses have tended to be ignored both by policy-makers and policy analysts. Nurses have not been militant or even very visible in policy terms. Nursing has had difficulty gaining access to policy and decision-making at both local and national levels (Clare, 1993). Nursing wants a voice in health care decision-making and wants responsibility, but those nurses with the credentials and backgrounds commensurate with the power desired are often not directly involved in health care delivery (Mauksch, 1980). Nursing and nursing values therefore have been marginal to the debates that have shaped UK health policy (Robinson *et al.*, 1992). Robinson and Strong (1987, 1988, 1989 and 1990) have ably documented this apparent invisibility. Nursing in the UK has currently lost its legitimate leadership position at all levels of decision-making in the health care system despite achieving a relative peak in power terms as a result of the 1974 NHS reorganization and the introduction of consensus management. At that time nurse managers took their place as equals of doctors, administrators and treasurers on the consensus management team.

In the reforms following the 1990 NHS and Community Care Act many health authorities see no place for nursing other than at operational level, although Trust boards are required to have an executive nurse member (Dean, 1990; Ham, 1992). Clinical directorates are almost exclusively headed up by doctors and nurses in primary health care settings, are being placed under the ever closer control of GPs despite the initial optimism surrounding possibilities for nurse-led primary care (DoH, 1989; NHSME, 1993).

Consequently, various pleas have been made for nurses to get 'political'; to begin to influence, rather than respond to and be the victim of, the political agenda (Maglacas, 1987; Smith, 1987; Salvage, 1997). Until the 1980s little attention was paid by most nurses to health policy formulation. Instead, apparently satisfied to focus primarily on the clinical aspects of care, nurses often shunned responsibility for taking part in health policy analysis and planning (Salvage 1985; Clay, 1987; Robinson, Gray and Elkan, 1992). Nevertheless, health policy affects nurses' daily work; it controls what practitioners can and cannot do and determines the type of care that patient's receive.

Health policy, however, has recently become a topic of increasing concern in nursing in the UK. Since the 1980s there has been an upsurge of interest in the 'politics of nursing' evidenced by the rising numbers of textbooks being published in the topic (Salvage, 1985; Clay, 1987; Fatchett, 1994). Nursing, particularly in the early 1980s, was seen as having a responsibility to work closely with public and private policy-makers in developing policies that constructively addressed health-related issues. This involvement in policy-making was perceived to be every bit as important a part of nursing's professional commitment, as providing the best possible nursing service to patients (Archer, 1983; Salvage, 1985; Clay, 1987). Since then, courses in health policy and policy-related topics have increasingly become integral parts of nursing curricula (UKCC, 1986; ENB, 1992). Yet there has been little coordinated theoretical development in this area in nursing (Robinson, 1991).

Nursing's invisibility and lack of political influence is not confined to the UK. Nurses the world over are undervalued and their views on vital social and health matters are often disregarded (Maglacas, 1987). As a result, the International Council of Nurses argued in 1987 that nursing was a valuable resource which should be actively utilized in health care policy and planning (Tierney, 1990; Chao, 1993). Nurses and nursing values must influence the making and implementation of health policy to enable nursing to make its optimal contribution to health services in all sectors and at all levels (Maglacas, 1987). Hence the development of a cadre of nurses who can competently and effectively analyse and influence the formulation of health policies to support nursing objectives is crucial.

Nurses in the USA have made some gains in this respect. On his election in 1992, President Clinton, whose mother was a nurse anaesthetist, openly sought advice on health care reform from the American Nurses' Association (ANA). Some of his key advisers on health are nurses and local branches of the ANA have representation and influence at the level of state administration. This success has been attributed to sophisticated political lobbying and a perceived sympathy for nursing ideals and values within Bill Clinton's camp. The American political system encourages an active role for pressure groups in lobbying Congress.

Current nursing values and theoretical frameworks

One of nursing's central values is to promote health. The WHO (1985) has even prompted nurses to consider themselves as the key professional group in this area. In Britain, the promotion of health is one of the nine nursing competencies necessary for first-level registration. Nevertheless, inequitable access to health and health care resources, economic impoverishment and unsafe physical surroundings inhibit health behaviours and threaten the well-being of countless people in the UK (Townsend and Davidson, 1992). Currently nurses are involved in health care systems that exclude or disadvantage large numbers of people who need care. The consequences of environmental devastation also threaten people's health on a global scale (Stevens and Hall, 1992).

Despite an emphasis on the core nursing values of holism and health, existent nursing theories do not address such global issues. Rather, they focus almost exclusively on individuals and their immediate surroundings (Peplau, 1952; Rogers, 1970; Newman, 1979; Johnson, 1980; King, 1981; Neuman, 1982; Roper, Logan and Tierney, 1983; Roy, 1984; Orem, 1985). Illustrating this point Cooke states:

> the ideological consensus within nursing focuses on the patient as an individual and on the nurse–patient relationship. Thus it fails to challenge the institutional context of nursing or address issues such as inequality which have a damaging effect on the delivery of nursing care. (Cooke, 1993; p. 1997)

By contrast, critical theory focuses on groups and communities and addresses the political and economic realities of the social order. People as individuals certainly can make changes to improve their well-being but a focus on individual responsibility, as emphasized by the 'New Right' (encapsulated by Thatcherism) and many nursing theorists, ends up blaming the victim and absolving government and society from any responsibility (Stevens and Hall, 1992). A district nursing student told me, for example, that she saw many similarities between Orem's theory of self-help and slogans such as 'on your bike' addressed to the unemployed by Conservative politicians such as Norman (now Lord) Tebbit in the mid-1980s. Frequently, nursing interventions are required in the many health problems caused by the oppression of ageism, sexism, racism and the unequal distribution of human rights (Kleffel, 1991). Therefore, a broader, more comprehensive view of persons, environments, health and the nature of nursing is necessary. Critical theory also views nurses from the standpoint of emancipative potential: that is a view which is in the interests of nurses rather than about nurses (De Marco, 1993). Kleffel (1991) suggested that when faced with problems and questions, such as those discussed above, which established theory cannot explain sufficiently, new investigations must begin that lead the profession towards a new theoretical basis for practice. Stevens (1989) heralds this new way of thinking and doing as:

> a powerful new lens, a frame of reference or interpretive scheme that is different from conventional nursing scholarship yet clearly in line with nursing's holistic perspective. (p. 61)

The future of nursing depends on nursing's ability to recognize the social, political and economic aspects of the environment as they affect nursing and health, and moreover a willingness to intervene for structural change. Critical theory offers a process that can empower nurses and nursing to undergo that change.

Critical theory with its focus on collectivity, consciousness-raising and discourse offers a legitimate and valuable means of conceptualizing nursing's current situation in health policy debates. As an associated research method, discourse analysis is suitable for pursuing further analysis and research in this area.

For example, health policy in the UK currently condones unsafe physical surroundings, oppressive social arrangements and poverty which effects the health of many people. Nursing values such as caring, equity and a sociopolitical model of health based on empowerment offer a potentially attractive alternative. Many authors have argued that nurses should join with vulnerable groups and, working together, expose these oppressive situations and take action for change (Stevens, 1989; Kleffel, 1991; Stevens and Hall, 1992; De Marco, 1993).

Critical theory is offered here as a means of illuminating the pathway to restructuring health care and enhancing, or perhaps even transforming, existing nursing theory. Critical theory contains the emancipatory goal of negotiating through authentic, culturally sensitive, communicative interaction the hope of a more ethically responsible community life (Ray, 1992).

For example, the research team at the Department of Education and Training/Patient Education Resource Centre at San Francisco's General Hospital sought to develop a patient education outreach effort at one of their satellite clinics, based on an empowerment model. The research team describe 'empowerment' as a participant-centred approach to planning, implementing and evaluating patient health education interventions. The approach fosters the building of skills, promotes patient and community competence and self-determination, helping to build community networks to support and augment health interventions begun in the clinical setting. The research team will facilitate the patients and their community to identify their own health concerns and propose specific educational interventions. At the same time practitioners will identify the relevant skills they need to acquire to support community empowerment (Personal Communication, 1996).

What is critical theory?

There is no single critical theory. Rather it informs and encompasses many perspectives, such as the German Frankfurt School, the liberation scholarship of developing countries and Black populations, feminist theory and lesbian and gay liberation studies. Key names associated with this school of thought are Adorno, Habermas, Bernstein. These perspectives share a common historical pattern of originating within resistance movements against such social conditions as fascism, colonisation, racism, sexism and prejudice against lesbians and gay men (Lather, 1986; Ray, 1992; Stevens and Hall, 1992).

Critical theorists are: 'united in their objectives: to empower the powerless and transform existing social inequalities and injustices' (McLaren, 1989, p. 160). Critical theory attempts to explain the social order in such a way that it itself becomes the catalyst which leads to the eventual transformation of the same social order (Fay, 1993). It assumes that society is marked by fundamental structural conflict and that this conflict produces deep suffering in all its members. All research, theory and practice are seen as political because they are intimately affected by the social, economic and political processes of society (Stevens and Hall, 1992). Critical theorists believe that one of the significant causes of oppression is the systematic ignorance or 'false consciousness' that oppressed members of society have about themselves and their society. If the oppressed – in this case nurses – came to have a different understanding of themselves they would be able to organize themselves into an effective group, with the power to alter their basic social arrangements and thus ease their suffering.

A colleague described to me a class she had been teaching to an all-female group of experienced nurse teachers, clinicians and managers. The aim of the class was to encourage students to look at their familiar worlds of home and work in new ways. One of the approaches she adopted was to draw up a reading list to encourage critical thinking during seminar presentation among the group. Prominent on the reading list were the writings and research studies of such feminist scholars as Oakley, Webb, Gilligan, Hall and Stevens. Two of the group took issue with my colleague for giving prominence to feminism and its analysis of oppression, which they saw as irrelevant. As White, middle-class senior nurse managers, they did not identify with the overtly oppressed groups described in some of the texts. Some months later, one of the critics was unexpectedly made redundant as a result of economic cutbacks in the community health trust where she worked. When her final assignment for the class was submitted, she had adopted a more sympathetic tone in her use of feminism as a theoretical device to analyse nursing's current situation. The cynic may attribute this change in tone to the student's need to please my colleague in order to obtain a 'good' grade. My colleague believed that feminism had given the student the means to analyse her situation of redundancy as being the result of economic policy rather than her own personal failure, thus giving her both an understanding of oppression (nursing jobs are dispensable) but also her liberation from an organization which did not value her.

Liberation from oppression is seen by critical theorists as an indispensable part of well-being and integrity, and is considered to result from a dialectical process of action and reflection. As originally formulated, especially by Marx, critical theory's primary intent centred on political revolutionary action (Ray, 1992).

Critical theories are not mere abstractions. Their basis is a living process created in the everyday struggles of a group of people. They are grounded in the historical context of a concrete oppressive condition experienced by a particular group. Thus they avoid the oppressive split between theory and practice, and academia and 'real' life, since critical theories affirm the oppressed as the subjects of their own struggle, rather than as objects of study or manipulation. Critical theory research is concerned with doing research with and for people rather than on people. It is not treated as a neutral, value-free process but as a supporting and questioning initiative (Reason and Rowan, 1981; Stevens and Hall, 1992). The core of critical theory scholarship therefore is the notion of emancipating people from conscious or unconscious constraints, to improve the lives of those involved and transform fundamental social structures and relationships (Ray, 1992).

Many examples of emancipation and transformation in peoples' lives can be identified from recent European history. Of interest are the writings of

Alexandra Kollontai, the only woman in Lenin's government following the 1917 Russian Revolution. Kollontai's writings demonstrate one of the central preoccupations of critical theorists and feminists: the interface between the political and the personal, in the social transformation of peoples' lives. Sheila Rowbottom (1978), commenting on Kollontai's work writes:

> She tried always to examine the gap between the official surface of things and the actuality within – and would not rest content with the easy formula that changes in the mode of production and external structure of work relations under communism would automatically create a new freedom and equality between the sexes ... She wanted complete equality between the sexes, realising that this necessitated big changes in the structure of the family, the organisation of domestic work and the economic position of women. (p.223)

As well as her political writings expressed in official pamphlets, Kollontai also wrote about women's dilemmas through popular literature. Critical readings of these texts, such as *Love of Worker Bees* and *A Great Love*, both written in 1922, are an interesting way to approach discourse analysis and to unravel issues of social control and oppression in peoples' lives.

Language as a form of oppression

Scholarship emerging from critical theory contains an important focus on language as a vehicle for social control and domination (Kruchs, 1990). Habermas (1979), for example, highlights the ways spoken language functions to reproduce relations of domination. In parallel yet different ways, feminism focuses on language as it intersects with consciousness in the creation of subjective and objective experiences of power and domination. Feminism, too, presents a model of critique and challenge that emphasizes consciousness-raising (Boxer, 1981; MacKinnon, 1982). Ideologies are seen as the underlying meaning systems which are subtly communicated in social interactions, including everyday conversation, news, media, entertainment, scientific writing, religious beliefs and so on (Parker, 1992; Stevens and Hall, 1992). These systems tend not to be immediately evident in everyday experience. Therefore a systematic critique of ideology is needed to uncover the power relations embedded in communication (Habermas, 1979).

Discourse

Central to critical theory is the concept of discourse. In written discourse, what the author intended and the meaning of the text may not necessarily coincide. However, an authentic critique of the ideology contained therein is possible (Hiraki, 1992). The core of such reflection is demystification: critical, penetrating questioning of the taken-for-granted aspects of particular circumstances. Through this process the oppressed can take what is unquestioned and tear away its veneer, renaming it from their own perspective (Stevens and Hall, 1992).

Systems of domination

In the social institution of nursing, pre-reflective practice rests on unquestioned assumptions about the world of health care. These are assumptions that have been laid down over years of inherited tradition. The political–economic order is defined consistently within these assumptions as being not one among many possible political arrangements, but rather as being a 'second nature'. (Bauman, 1976). While these tacit theses usually go unnoticed, they become visible and objectively real when their legitimacy is challenged and it becomes recognized that the established order is only one possible way of constructing reality. This realization involves the recognition that the established order is maintained by power relations, or relations of domination (Thompson, 1987). Such consciousness-raising involves recognizing and helping others to recognize the social, political and economic impediments to equality. It also includes conceiving how to take action to change oppressive conditions (Stevens and Hall, 1992).

Critical scholarship in nursing

Critical theory has been described as currently marginal in nursing (Thompson, 1987) and certainly there are relatively few articles and books currently available in British nursing libraries which explore this approach. Consequently this discussion draws extensively from Thompson's (1987) work. Cooke (1993) argued that the older human science perspectives have been instrumental in coercing people and creating the 'disciplinary power' of modern society. Nursing academics, she asserted, have a choice between acting as social critics or accepting the 'protective bonds of patronage' and allying themselves with the forces of domination. Critical theory potentially opens up a whole new world for nursing through its systematic uncovering and critique of domination. It challenges contemporary perspectives on nursing and definitions of health and well-being. Critical scholars in nursing can provide a systematic and thorough critique of the hidden sources of coercion, power-over and domination that are embedded in the everyday 'lived experience' (Thompson, 1987). Critical scholars ask demystifying questions such as:

How have oppressive conditions developed over time? Who has access to resources? Whose interests have been served as a result of the way things are? (Stevens and Hall, 1992, p. 5)

The process of critical scholarship thus is one that rests on reflection and insight or consciousness-raising, where we comes to see ourselves through the reconstruction of our own self-formative process (Freire, 1972). Critical scholarship thus exposes the ways in which the self – in this case nursing – has been formed (or deformed) through the influence of coercive power relations. Once nurses become aware of and see through these power relations, the power relations lose power.

Importantly for nurses, the critique of domination can be experienced in ways characterized by joy and the pleasure of freedom. But paradoxically, it can also be experienced in ways that are full of pain and disorientation, as more and more practical assumptions and values are brought into question (Thompson, 1987). Such consciousness-raising is an act of transforming the social world. Through the process of exposing distorted power relations, critical scholarship forms the basis for a continuation of emancipatory and empowering work. That work includes the development of new language, new meanings and new social practices and hence the transformation of social institutions that have been oppressive (Thompson, 1987). Empowerment is an actual as well as a perceived sense of power, an observable effect on sociopolitical structures as well as subjective personal experience. Empowerment, therefore, within critical theory, involves material issues of resources and their control within a wider social context and requires political activity (Katz, 1984).

Drawing on critical theory, Smith and Agard (1997) describe and comment on frontline care given by a public health nurse in a US inner city. They note many factors which affect her work, not least the tense economic atmosphere of recession and competition which pare public services and benefits to the bone. Only the most needy and complex clients find their way on to her case load. The vignettes describe an African–American man with AIDS recovering from a traumatic hospitalization and a young woman with a new baby, also African–American, who is undergoing rehabilitation for a drug habit. Part of the nurse's job is to become a 'broker' by which she connects her clients to the voluntary and public services they need. Like teachers and social workers, she tries to close the gap between what is needed and what can be provided but she controls neither the demand for the services nor the resources to meet those demands. Administrators make decisions based on financial and organizational criteria. The views and experiences of the direct service providers, like the public health nurse, are rarely involved in these decisions nor incorporated into the criteria on which they are made.

These vignettes illuminate many critical theory tenets about nursing such as theory is inextricably linked to practice and care occurs within a social context. Nursing is turning to critical theory in a quest to gain in-depth understanding of the dynamics of nursing's social and political context (Ray, 1992). Critical theory enables the institutionalized power relations and relations of domination in the social reality of nursing to be challenged (Thompson, 1987).

Nurses are increasingly becoming sensitized to the power relations anchored in race, gender and class (Thompson, 1987). In the vignettes, for example, race, gender and class are in evidence. It is no accident the public health nurse is a woman, as are the majority of nurses, teachers and social workers in the USA and Western Europe. It is now recognized particularly among the feminist literature that the type of work traditionally done by women because of its domestic associations is often underrated and poorly valued. Client status is also associated with how work is rated and valued. Services for groups perceived as having low status, such as the elderly, the disabled and mentally ill, for example, are traditionally referred to as the 'Cinderella' services. In the USA and increasingly in Britain, the community or public health nursing services tend to serve those who are marginalized because of their class, employment status, race, gender and sexual orientation. The individuals in the vignettes, for example, were suffering from AIDS and drug addiction which are stigmatized, victim-blaming conditions.

Working with stigmatized clients may also affect the status of those working with them. Nurses who work with marginalized clients, particularly those who are perceived as bringing their illnesses and conditions on themselves, may find they are also marginalized and undervalued. Their work is seen to be less useful than those nurses who specialize in acute care. Furthermore, research informed by critical perspectives reveals how Black nurses were specifically recruited to undertake lower level training and channelled into Cinderella specialities (Baxter, 1988; King's Fund, 1990; Maslin-Prothero, 1992; Beishon, Virdee and Hagell, 1995). Their promotion prospects were also poorer than those of their White counterparts.

Critical theory thus can help nursing to address the multiple sources of power and domination in health care for both client and worker; to focus on the politics of consciousness and the subjective experience of powerlessness; and to tackle the inherited social structures and practices that comprise externally imposed sources of domination (Thompson, 1987). Critical theory also aims to facilitate nursing emancipation from these oppressive social systems so that nursing in its turn can help patients and clients secure improved conditions. Critical theory brings to consciousness the patriarchal, economic and medical models that support authoritarianism and suppress human caring values. It fosters self-consciousness about existing social, political, technologic and economic conditions. Critical theory therefore can contribute to reforming health care to include equal roles for nursing with other health care professionals, as a means of improving the moral character of community life (Ray, 1992).

Gadow (1980) argued that:

> The direction in which nursing develops will determine whether the profession draws closer to the medical model, with its commitment to science, technology and cure; reverts to historical nursing models with their essentially intuitive approaches; or creates a new philosophy that sets contemporary nursing apart from both traditional nursing and modern medicine. (p. 101)

In summary, then, critical theory can show nurses how to 'reweave the fabric' of their social world, how to envision and construct a coherent political base for positive practical action through giving nursing a voice and a role in the construction of a more egalitarian world (Thompson, 1987). Critical theory and discourse analysis are an empowering combination and a case will be advanced for putting them on the nursing research agenda.

Critical theory and discourse analysis – an empowering combination

Because of its illuminatory and emancipatory powers, discourse analysis is a research method which is congruent with the theoretical perspective of critical theory. As previously mentioned, there is a minimal amount of nursing research using this method. One way to remedy this situation is to describe the breadth of method involved in discourse analysis, the tools and techniques utilized in the research process and to consider some of its advantages and disadvantages. Some research examples using discourse analysis are presented.

Critical theory which underpins discourse analysis holds a dynamic and shifting view of reality, acknowledging the intrinsic subjectivity and biases of all forms of research inquiry (Thompson, 1987; Cooke, 1993). It views knowledge and understanding as a process rather than an outcome; research is done in collaboration with participants (Stanley and Wise, 1993).The position of the researcher and the researched are as equals and research findings are seen as intrinsic. Critical theory welcomes action (Freire, 1972; Thompson, 1987; Cooke, 1993).

Robinson and Elkan (1989) have identified the need for research which uncovers the 'important information': that is, research that gets behind the description and begins in the first instance to develop explanations for why health care exists as it is, and in the second, to discuss how change could be accomplished. Clare (1993) re-emphasized Robinson and Elkan's request, stating that:

> Nurses collectively must discover processes and act to transform the social structures which support the sources of power limiting nursing autonomy in every area of nursing education and practice. Perhaps then a 'revolution' of both nursing practice and nursing education could take place for the benefit of our clients. (p. 1037)

Discourse analysis offers a social account of subjectivity by attending to the linguistic resources by which the sociopolitical realm is produced and reproduced (Burnam and Parker, 1993). It involves an attention to the ways in which language and other representational systems such as art and music do more than reflect what they represent. Meanings are seen to be multiple and shifting rather than unitary and fixed. Discourse analysis provokes a deconstruction of the 'truths' we take as given (Macnaghten, 1993). It requires a self-conscious attention to account, presentation and context in the illumination of power relations in society and as such can be used to inform political practice and struggles (Burnam and Parker, 1993). It highlights the social processes which participate in the maintenance of structures of oppression. Discourse analysis, underpinned by critical theory, therefore appears to offer a route to Clare's 'revolution'.

What is discourse analysis?

In reviewing the literature relating to discourse analysis there seems to be some inconsistency in the way terms are used. Historically, documentary analysis seems to have been the most commonly used term up until the 1970s when it appears to have been replaced with discourse analysis, linked to Continental philosophy and imbued with notions of consciousness-raising, reflection and emancipation.

In terms of the contemporary social scientific analysis of documents, the work of Thomas and Znaniecki is credited as having an early and seminal influence (Billig, 1988; Parker, 1992; Jupp and Norris, 1993). Documentary analysis has been used in a wide range of disciplines including social psychology, social anthropology, political science, sociology, criminology and history.

Documentary analysis has a positivistic heritage and content analysis was thus typically concerned initially with the explicit content and superficial meaning rather than with deeper layers of meaning (Shipman, 1997). Content analysis within the positivist paradigm assumed that there were attributes, attitudes and values relating to individuals represented unambiguously in the manifest contents of documents. Many studies of political values were undertaken in the US using this method in the 1940s and 1950s (Jupp and Norris, 1993). Similarly sociologists and social anthropologists have used documents as expressions of social and cultural values.

In the 1960s the interpretative tradition in sociology argued that social phenomena were socially constructed and criticized the positivist approach to documentary analysis, arguing that it ignored the effects of normative rules on the communicator and the interpretation of the analyst (Jupp and Norris, 1993).

The newest perspective on discourse analysis – the critical paradigm – encourages a focus on the relationship between documents and social structure, class relations, social control, social order, ideology and power (Bhavnani, 1990). Foucault (1982 cited in Plummer, 1983), for example, highlights how discourse analysis can reveal the mechanisms by which power is exercised. The central concepts and emphases of the critical paradigm raise important questions which can be examined via documents and texts, namely a concern with analysis at a societal and social structural level; an emphasis on conflicts between social groupings and the dynamics of struggles between them; an accent on power and control in the relationships between social groupings; an interest in ideology as a means through which existing structures and social arrangements are legitimated and maintained; a commitment to 'not taking for granted' what is said; and finally a commitment to changing the existing order (Jupp and Norris, 1993).

Wright and Shore (1995) demonstrate the use of anthropology to critically analyse the disciplinary limitations of policy studies in the spirit of 'not taking [anything] for granted'. Their critique resonates with discourse analysis. They suggest that the convention within policy studies to treat policies 'as instruments of governance: rational, non-theoretical and goal-orientated tools that provide the most efficient means to obtaining certain desired ends' (p.28), serves to disassociate them from morality, ideology and politics. It follows therefore that political decision-making on the part of governments can be objectified, which in turn absolves them from assuming responsibility for both their policies and actions.

Wright and Shore draw on the following example from a recent incident in British politics to illustrate their argument. In the Conservative government's 1993 'back to basics' policy 'ministers emphasised their commitment to a political philosophy based on so-called "traditional family values" and launched a crusade against the immorality of single mothers and absentee fathers' (p.29). The initiative backfired when it was revealed that a junior government minister, Tim Yeo, had fathered two children during an extra-marital affair. Yeo, however, 'When talking about single parents as the subjects of policy, clearly did not include his mistress and his own adulterous circumstances and was annoyed when journalists and commentators did so'. Equally revealing for Wright and Shore were Prime Minister John Major's attempts to defend Yeo's behaviour as 'a foolish indiscretion' whereas the single mothers were 'guilty of "bad behaviour" '. Clearly, Mr Yeo did not see his 'own behaviour as having anything to do with the policy classification his government was imposing on others'. Thus, 'policy often functions as a vehicle for distancing the policy authors from the intended objects of policy. Equally, perhaps, it serves as a mechanism for disguising the identity of decision-makers' (p.29).

Discourse analysis is typically associated with socialist/liberation approaches to research. However, Burnam and Parker (1993) highlight how the political Right have 'hijacked' discourses. Using race as an example, they show that a move away from biological theories of racial inferiority to discourses which support notions of cultural difference and pluralism have been used to justify an association between difference and 'inevitable' conflict which can only be solved through repatriation. For example, Enoch Powell, who ironically was involved in recruiting West Indians for the NHS (Bilton *et al.*, 1987,) delivered inflammatory speeches in the 1960s, in which the British public were warned that if immigration was allowed to go unchecked, bloodshed would result as indigenous and immigrant communities competed for scarce resources (Butler and Pinto-Duschinsky, 1971). For Powell, the only solution was to send the latter 'home' to their countries of origin.

Discourse analysis in nursing

Delacour (1991) comments that until recently nursing has been 'spoken' by others and that the gap between professional nursing discourse and the dominant social construction of nursing is enormous. Nurses are only now beginning to investigate discourses and a brief review of the extent of the available literature is detailed below.

Weiss (1985) was committed to collaborative models of care based on a biopyschosocial approach as a means of allowing consumers and nurses a greater role in health care. She set up a study using experimental and control groups to determine whether or not a monthly discussion concerning health care relationships among nurses, doctors and consumers influenced their collaborative beliefs and behaviour over a two-year period. No particular theoretical framework was identified. All participants completed the Management of Differences Exercise, the Multidimensional Health Locus of Control Scales and the Health Expectations Index at the start and finish of the study. Perhaps unsurprisingly in view of the current dominance of medicine and medical values in health care, but sadly nevertheless, the results suggested that the experimental group were less sure of the value of collaborative models of care and more sure about the doctors' positive effect on health status than the control group, thus indicating that the ongoing discourse may have enhanced rather than reduced the traditional authority and power of the doctor.

Thompson (1985), in positive contrast to Weiss' rather negative findings, argued that nursing is reaching an intellectual maturity as evidenced in its interest in looking critically through discourse analysis at the way it practises science. She called this 'self-consciousness' and asserted that nurse researchers have become aware of the biases and prejudices inherent in nursing research programmes.

Elliot (1989) argued that nursing is systematically silenced at all levels and in all types of communication. She identified that historically nurses have learned and used the language of medicine which remains the 'official' language of health care. She suggested that what nurses talk about

– that is, the pragmatics of their discourse – is not considered official or noteworthy by the men's world of medicine and health care finance. Thus she emphazised that nurses are controlled by patriarchy at home, through the hospital and the state. She dismissed innovations such as nursing diagnosis, which some authors have heralded as a means of empowering nursing, arguing that its tendency toward exclusive use by graduates in nursing simply reinforces the race and class divisions of women in nursing. The solution to this silencing, Elliot suggests, is in communicating the work of all nurses through a visible and accurate discourse, understandable to all nurses and proclaimed loudly. She also requested a unity in the voice of nursing and a general acknowledgement among nurses that practice is the most prestigious work of nursing.

Hiraki (1992) investigated the language used to describe, explain and interpret the concept of the nursing process in four introductory textbooks. She used a critical theory framework to reinterpret the ways in which such discourse constructs the social–historical reality of nurses. Themes related to tradition, rationality and power relationships were explicated. The meanings disclosed from these texts provide understandings about how nurses interpret their professional autonomy and how normative structures inform what constitutes authority and responsibility in research, education and practice.

Johnson (1993), using discourse analysis in combination with ethnography, studied nurse practitioner–patient interactions with a view to understanding the positive outcomes of nurse practitioner care. She showed that the nurse practitioner's discourse differed from that of the doctor's and thus identified a distinct nursing perspective on care. This perspective was characterized by a focus on the patient's perceived concern rather than their medical problem, the use of a shared language and partnership. In her conclusions, Johnson urged nurse practitioners to consider how such contextual factors as power, gender and ideology provide the subtext for medical domination in health care and suggested that such reflection may help nurses to have their voices heard and enable consumers to access nursing as opposed to medical care.

Ryan and Porter (1993) examined the sex of contributors to the *Journal of Advanced Nursing* and found that men contributed 45.1 per cent of the UK-based writers in contrast to 5.5 per cent of the North American contributors. Similarly they discovered that 46.1 per cent of the contributors to *Senior Nurse* were men. Therefore, despite their relatively low numbers in the profession, men's contributions in mainstream nursing journals have reached a level where they have great influence over how nursing conceptualizes itself. This male control of nursing discourse matters very much, as language is of crucial importance in the way we think about the world and dominance over discourse is one of the fundamental bases of social and occupational power (Ryan and Porter, 1993).

Masterson (1994) selected primary nursing as a case study to demonstrate Bachrach and Baratz's (1962) concept of non-decision-making in action and the complex relationship between health policy and the construction of nursing. In her analysis she explored how primary nursing achieved such rapid success as an innovation, growing from a mere whisper in the nursing journals in the late 1970s, to practically being enshrined in statute with the inclusion of 'named nursing' in the Patient's Charter in 1991. In her conclusions she argued for an in-depth analysis of contemporary nursing and health policy literature using discourse analysis within the framework of critical theory to help nurses demystify, delegitimate and deconstruct established values and institutions through analysing the discourses that create and maintain oppression. Such an analysis would aim to identify the values expressed in these discourses and, from that illumination, raise awareness among nurses of their current powerlessness and their future potential, thereby challenging the existing order in health care and enabling nursing to make its optimal contribution to health. Similarly, Mary Finch (1991) identified the rise of Thatcherism and a change in social values as important contributory factors to the rise of primary nursing.

Swann and Ussher (1995) used a discourse analytic approach to take on board the social construction of pre-menstrual syndrome (PMS) and women's subjective experience of the condition. They felt such an approach acknowledged the complexity of PMS as a phenomenon and took account of its relationship to female identity and to the social context of the female reproductive body.

From the preceding review, it can be concluded that discourse analysis provides a wonderful opportunity for nursing to combine knowledge for practice with broader goals of emancipation. No other method blends successfully the almost contrary needs as demonstrated by the vignettes, for an understanding of nursing and its relationships on a micro-level coupled with an insightful consideration of nursing's interactions with social institutions and the social order itself.

Part 2: Methodological issues

Despite a growing body of literature about discourse analysis *per se* and significant amounts of literature which describe the results of such analyses across many diverse fields, there appears to a dearth of literature about the 'how to' of the process. Consequently there seems to be a confusing proliferation of brands of discourse analysis, all with multiple origins, each of which involve different emphases or levels and styles of analysis. Some of this ambiguity is perhaps intentional and desirable. Burnam and Parker (1993), both psychologists, argued that it is very difficult to speak of discourse analysis as a single unitary entity: 'as this would blur together approaches subscribing to specific and different philosophical frameworks'

(p. 3). All approaches are united however by a common attention to the significance and structuring effects of language, and are associated with interpretive and reflective styles of analysis.

Literature as a source for discourse analysis

Documentary sources offer a potentially rich source of evidence which avoids many of the snags associated with research involving obtrusion into human activity (Shipman, 1997). Nursing journals and publications form part of professional nursing discourse: that is, the set of values, meanings and beliefs that are important to the profession and that are implicated in some way with the structure of the institutions of health care and health policy-making (Chapman, 1988; Parker, 1992). Foucault (1972) argued that discourses and practices could be treated as if they were the same thing, as discourses systematically form the objects of which they speak. 'Discourses construct representations of the world which have a reality almost as coercive as gravity' (Parker, 1992, p.8), 'and discourses therefore are structured around and reproduce power relations' (Turner, 1987).

For example, little attention has been paid to the ideological and political issues embedded in the nursing literature yet the values expressed in such literature should not only reflect nurses' reality but also have the potential power to affect readers' thoughts and actions. The values expressed inform and reflect practice and many authors such as Hiraki (1992) have argued that such a reinterpretation of nursing literature from a critical perspective is needed desperately, to make explicit the cultural and political meanings hidden in the taken-for-granted metaphors which are used to describe the nature of nursing.

The analytic process

Critical theory asserts that all forms of social reality have a peculiarly human and socially constructed nature (Macnaghten, 1993): that is, knowledge is irretrievably connected to a reality – produced, bounded and sustained by human meanings and constructions. Language therefore can actually produce a social reality as well as describe it. Hence the aim of discourse analysis is to unravel the processes through which discourse is constructed and the consequences of these constructions.

Parker (1992) identifies several stages that the researcher should take. Content analysis is part of this process. Content analysis refers to a means of summarizing, standardizing and comparing or otherwise systematically transforming already existing data (Smith, 1975). Content analysis should contain both a latent and manifest dimension. Manifest analysis is where explicit words, terms and phrases are identified which can be taken as an indicator of values. Latent analysis involves identifying the code and major thrust or intent of a discourse, and therefore the implicit values being expressed. That is, it goes beyond what is written or said directly and infers meaning (Field and Morse, 1985).

Discourse research aims to strike a critical distance from language and the researcher must therefore engage in reflexivity (Parker, 1992). Consequently as the analysis proceeds it is necessary metaphorically to 'step back' a number of times to make sense of the values picked out and the interpretations and conclusions drawn. The first step is to describe the meanings of the texts. All connotations, allusions and implications should then be explored. Throughout it is important to question who the discourse is addressing and what the readers are expected to do once addressed.

Levy and Guttman (1985) asserted that both quantitative and qualitative data can be derived from documentary sources. They suggested that the strength of importance or feeling ascribed to a value can be quantified by simply counting the number of times it occurred. Kovach (1993) also favours quantitative analysis, arguing that such a process assists in the generalizability of findings. She does sound a note of caution, however, asserting that the researcher must reassure themselves that frequency of occurrence is really a basis for making such inferences.

Parker (1992) indicated that all the discourses contain, uphold, and rest on other discourses. Contradictions may well be identified between the different ways values are described. Any interrelationships between discourses and their suggested consequences should be explored thoroughly. Consequently, other texts should be referred to as the need arises to elaborate the discourses as they appear. Attempts should be made to locate and consider the discourses within their temporal, social and historical contexts. Hence how and where discourses emerge should be identified and any changes therein described. Institutions should be distinguished which are reinforced or attacked by various discourses. Similarly categories of person should be isolated as gaining and losing from the employment of certain discourses to endeavour to establish who would want to promote, and who would want to dissolve, such discourses. Finally the researcher should aim to show how particular discourses connect with other discourses; and the power relationships involved.

The minutiae and pragmatics of the process

Before beginning a discourse analysis the researcher should explicate her own values. Each source should then be considered thoroughly with a suspicious eye. As the sources are examined, questions should be continually asked of them like: 'Why was this said and not that? Why these words, and how do these words fit with different ways of talking about the world?' (Parker, 1992). Billig (1988) emphasizes the need to look for both implicit and explicit themes. Once themes have been explicated, they should be organized under categories. Often categories will not be mutually exclusive of each other, nor will each of the themes. Ease of analysis and appropriateness should be the bases for developing categories and themes. Finally, discourse analysis is hard work. It is extremely labour-intensive and takes time to learn and develop the skills of analysis (Gill, 1993).

Ensuring reliability, validity and rigour in discourse analysis

There is some tension and disagreement among discourse analysts regarding reliability, validity and rigour. Polit and Hungler (1995) argued that the key issue concerning validity in research, whatever the method, is whether or not the data gathered by the researcher reflect reality. A danger inherent in discourse analysis is that researchers will simply verify their own preconceptions (Billig, 1988). Hence some proponents suggest key questions to be answered with regard to reliability and validity in discourse analysis. For example, would another researcher extract the same information from the available documents? Has enough care been taken to ensure that superfluous information has not been taken as being central? Would other researchers have interpreted the material differently? How far can the information that has been extracted be generalized? (Parker, 1992; Shipman, 1997).

As a measure of reliability they suggest that the researcher could ask someone totally unconnected with the research to analyse 'blind' a piece of data that she had already analysed. However, Potter and Wetherell (1987) note that this could end up merely describing and confirming common sense. Alternatively, other authors argue that inherent in the nature of discourse analysis is the assumption that different people will give different slants on the discourse depending on whether or not they stand to benefit from it (Parker, 1992).

Certainly it seems reasonable to suggest that by the researcher explicating her own values before beginning the analysis, bias could be lessened by ensuring a reduced tendency to focus on superfluous material because it fits with the researcher's own assumptions. This approach is similar to the technique of bracketing used by phenomenologists.

Lincoln and Guba (1985) offer an interesting alternative approach to assess the rigour of research of the qualitative type. They suggest credibility, applicability, consistency and confirmability as alternative conceptualizations of reliability and validity. Credibility occurs when the researcher immediately identifies herself with the experiences described by another person. Applicability relates to the findings 'fitting' into contexts outside the study situation. Consistency questions the ability of another researcher to follow the thinking, logic, decisions and methods used by the original investigator. And confirmability involves an audit of the process and the product.

Lather (1986), in a similar vein, attempts to reconceptualize validity within the context of openly ideological research using 'data credibility checks' based on a consideration of triangulation, construct validity, face validity and catalytic validity. Triangulation dictates the use of multiple sources of data, methods and theoretical schemes which, he argues, should lead to data trustworthiness in that both 'counter patterns and convergences' within data can be checked out. Construct validity can be evaluated by means of reflexivity, a key concept of critical theory. This means that the researcher should systematically report how decisions were taken at all steps in the research process and how the researcher herself influenced the content and process of the research. Face validity is assessed by 'member checks' or having research participants 'recycle' the analysis and then refining it according to their reactions. This would be difficult to accomplish in discourse analysis using widely available sources with a huge range of contributors. The notion of catalytic validity relates to the change-promoting aims of critical research and involves questioning whether or not the research has been successful in stimulating change.

Nevertheless, limitations acknowledged, I would concur with Gill (1993) that discourse analysis offers both a practical, systematic and theoretically coherent way of analysing a whole variety of texts in order to understand ideology and its effects on nursing.

Some conclusions

In the preceding discussions, through a case study of nursing and health policy, I have outlined the potential contribution of discourse analysis, particularly underpinned with critical theory, as a useful tool to both shape and operationalize the nursing research agenda. Like the NHS itself, the current NHS research agenda and the structures resulting from it, which shape and control nursing research, are the outcome of governmental values and the negotiation and bargaining of powerful groups such as medicine and commerce. Discourse analysis within the critical paradigm can reveal the mechanisms by which such power is exercised. Nursing research is currently seen as fragmented, devoid of a clear strategy and vision, and isolated from the wider body of research in the health arena (Traynor and Rafferty, 1997). But nurses are in an ideal position to identify health and social needs and must therefore take an active role in policy formulation and implementation in relation to research to be able to truly develop practice for the benefit of humanity (Ehrenfeld, Bergmen and Krulik, 1993; Traynor and Rafferty, 1997).

Critical scholarship provides an avenue for nursing to develop this attitude change or conscientization as it encourages a broad, comprehensive view of persons, health, environment and the nature of nursing (Ray, 1992; Stevens and Hall, 1992). It focuses on the politics of consciousness and the subjective experience of powerlessness, thus addressing domination and oppression (Thompson, 1987). Dominant ideologies are subtly communicated in the discourses of conversation, academic publications, policy documents and so on. Policy documents and texts are therefore forms of data which can play a vital part in research (Plummer, 1983; Jupp and Norris, 1993). Discourse analysis enables the investigation of the relationship between documents and social structures, class relations, social control, social order, ideology and power (Bhavnani, 1990). Such research has the potential to make an important contribution to the development of practice and the empowerment of nursing.

References

Archer S E (1983) Playing the political game. *Nursing Times* 6 April: 51–5.

Bachrach P and Baratz M S (1962) The two faces of power. *American Political Science Review* 56: 947–52.

Bauman Z (1976) *Toward a Critical Sociology: an Essay on Common-sense and Emancipation*. Routledge & Kegan Paul, London.

Baxter C (1988) *The Black Nurse: an Endangered Species*. National Extension College, Cambridge.

Beardshaw V (1992) Prospects for nursing. In Beck E, Lonsdale S, Newman S and Patterson D *In the Best of Health? The Status and Future of Healthcare in the UK.* Chapman & Hall, London: 103–22.

Beer S H (1969) *Modern British Politics*, 2nd edn. Faber, London.

Beishon S, Virdee S and Hagell A (1995) *Nursing in a Multi-ethnic NHS*. Policy Studies Institute, London.

Bhavnani K (1990) What's power got to do with it? Empowerment and social research. In Parker I and Shotter J (eds) *Deconstructing Social Psychology*. Routledge, London.

Billig M (1988) Methodology and scholarship in understanding ideological explanation. In Antaki C (ed.) *Analysing Everyday Explanation: a Casebook of Methods*. Sage, London: 199–215.

Bilton T, Bonnett K, Jones P, Stanworth M, Sheard K and Webster A (1987) *Introductory Sociology*, 2nd edn. Macmillan, Basingstoke.

Boxer M (1981) For and about women: the theory and practice of women's studies in the United States. In Keohane N, Rosaldo M and Gelpi B (eds) *Feminist Theory: a Critique of Ideology*. University of Chicago Press, Chicago: 237–71.

Buchan J (1991) Assessing the cost of nursing. *Nursing Standard* 6(4): 40.

Burnam E and Parker I (1993) (eds) *Discourse Analytic Research: Repertoires and Readings of Texts in Action*. Routledge, London.

Butler D and Pinto-Duschinsky M (1971) *The British General Election of 1970*. Macmillan, Basingstoke.

Chao Y Y (1993) Developing national health policy in Taiwan. *International Nursing Review* 40(6): 171–87.

Chapman G E (1988) Reporting therapeutic discourse in a therapeutic community. *Journal of Advanced Nursing* 13: 255–64.

Clare J (1993) A challenge to the rhetoric of emancipation: recreating a professional culture. *Journal of Advanced Nursing* 18(7): 1033–8.

Clay T (1987) *Nurses, Power and Politics*. Heinemann, London.

Cooke H (1993) Boundary work in the nursing curriculum: the case of sociology. *Journal of Advanced Nursing* 18(12): 1990–8.

Dean D (1990) Where has all the power gone? *Nursing Standard* 4(48), 22 August: 17–19.

Delacour S (1991) The construction of nursing: ideology, discourse and representation. In Gray G and Pratt R (eds) *Towards a Discipline of Nursing*. Churchill Livingstone, Melbourne.

De Marco R (1993) Mentorship: a feminist critique of current research. *Journal of Advanced Nursing* 18(8): 1242–50.

Department of Health (1989) *Working for patients*. HMSO, London.

Department of Health (1992) *Report of the Taskforce on the Strategy for Research in Nursing, Midwifery and Health Visiting*. HMSO, London.

Ehrenfeld M, Bergman R and Krulik T (1993) Final requirement for a Master's degree in nursing: health care policy and its implementation. *Journal of Nursing Management* 1: 143–7.

Elliot E A (1989) The discourse of nursing: a case of silencing. *Nursing and Health Care* 10(10): 539–43.

English National Board for Nursing, Midwifery and Health Visiting (1992) *Higher Award*. ENB, London.

Fatchett A (1994) *Politics, Policy and Nursing*. Ballière Tindall, London.

Fay B (1993) The elements of critical social science: 33–6. In Hammersley M *Social Research: Philosophy, Politics and Practice*. Sage, London.

Field P and Morse J (1985) *Nursing research: the Application of Qualitative Approaches*. Croom Helm, Beckenham.

Finch M (1991) The steady advance of a revolution. *Nursing Times* 87(17): 67–8.

Foucault M (1972) *The Archaeology of Knowledge*. Tavistock, London.

Freire P (1972) *Pedagogy of the Oppressed*. Penguin Books, London.

Gadow S (1980) Existential advocacy: philosophical foundations of nursing. In Spiker S F and Gadow S, (eds) *Nursing: Ideas and Images Opening Dialogue with the Humanities*. Springer-Verlag, New York: 79–101.

Gill R (1993) Justifying injustice: broadcasters' accounts of inequality in radio. In Burnam E and Parker I (eds) *Discourse Analytic Research: Repertoires and Readings of Texts in Action*. Routledge, London: 75–93.

Habermas J (1979) *Communication and the Evolution of Society*, McCarthy T (trans). Beacon Press, Boston.

Ham C (1992) *Health Policy in Britain: the Politics and Organisation of the National Health Service*, 3rd edn. Macmillan, Basingstoke.

Hiraki A (1992) Tradition, rationality and power in introductory nursing textbooks: a critical hermeneutics study. *Advances in Nursing Science* 14(3): 1–12.

Johnson D (1980) The behavioural system model for nursing. In Riehl J P and Roy C (eds) *Conceptual Models for Nursing Practice*, 2nd edn. Appleton-Century-Crofts, New York.

Johnson R (1993) Nurse practitioner–patient discourse: uncovering the voice of nursing in primary care practice. *Scholarly Inquiry for Nursing Practice* 7(3): 143–57.

Jupp V and Norris C (1993) Traditions in documentary analysis: 37–51. In Hammersley M *Social Research: Philosophy, Politics and Practice*. Sage, London.

Katz R (1984) Empowerment and synergy: expanding the community's healing resources. *Prevention in Human Services* 3: 201–6.

King I (1981) *A Theory of Nursing*. John Wiley, Chichester.

King's Fund (1990) *Racial equality: the nursing profession*. Equal Opportunity Task Force Occasional Paper, 6, King's Fund, London.

Kleffel D (1991) Rethinking the environment as a domain of nursing knowledge. *Advances in Nursing Science* 14(1): 40–51.

Kovach C R (1993) Development and testing of the autobiographical coding tool. *Journal of Advanced Nursing* 18: 669–74.

Kruchs S (1990) *Situation and Human Existence: Freedom, Subjectivity and Society*. Unwin Hyman, London.

Lather P (1986) Research as praxis. *Harvard Educational Review* 556(3): 257–77.

Levy S and Guttman L (1985) Faceted cross-cultural analysis of some true core social values. In Carter D (ed.) *Facet Theory: Approaches to Social Research*. Springer-Verlag, New York.

Lincoln Y S and Guba E G (1985) *Naturalistic Inquiry*. Sage, Newbury Park.

Liss P E (1993) *Health Care Need*. Avebury, Aldershot.

MacKinnon C (1982) Feminism, Marxism, method and the state: an agenda for theory. *Signs* 7: 515–44.

McLaren P (1989) *Life in Schools: an Introduction to Critical Pedagogy in the Foundations of Education*. Longman, London.

Macnaghten, P (1993) Discourses of nature: argumentation and power. In Burnam E and Parker I (eds) *Discourse Analytic Research: Repertoires and Readings of Texts in Action*. Routledge, London: 52–74.

Maglacas (1987) Reported in News. *Journal of Advanced Nursing* 13: 289.

Maslin-Prothero S (1992) Minority ethnic women and nursing. *Nursing Standard* 7(8): 25–8.

Masterson A (1994) An exploration of the values of British nursing and the values enshrined in the UK health policy: a research proposal. MN Dissertation, University of Wales, Cardiff.

Mauksch I (1980) Faculty practice: a professional imperative. *Nurse Educator* 5: 21–4.

National Health Service Management Executive (1993) *New World, New Opportunities. Nurse in Primary Health Care*. NHSME, London.

Neuman B (1982) *The Neuman Systems Model: Application to Nursing Education and Practice*. Appleton-Century-Crofts, Norwalk.

Newman M (1979) *Theory Development in Nursing*. Davis, Philadelphia.

Orem D (1985) *Nursing: Concepts of Practice*. McGraw-Hill, New York.

Parker I (1992) *Discourse Dynamics: Critical Analysis for Social and Individual Psychology*. Routledge, London.

Peplau H (1952) *Interpersonal Relations in Nursing*. Pitman, New York.

Plummer K (1983) *Documents of Life*. Allen & Unwin, London.

Polit D F and Hungler B P (1995) *Nursing Research: Principles and Methods*, 5th edn. J B Lippincott, Philadephia.

Potter, J and Wetherell M (1987) *Discourse and Social Psychology: Beyond Attitudes and Behaviour*. Sage, London.

Ray M A (1992) Critical theory as a framework to enhance nursing science. *Nursing Science Quarterly* 5(3) Fall: 98–101.

Reason P and Rowan J (eds) (1981) *Human Inquiry: a Sourcebook of New Paradigm Research*. John Wiley, Chichester.

Robinson J (1991) Power, politics and policy analysis in nursing. In Perry A and Jolley M (eds) *Nursing a Knowledge Base for Practice*. Edward Arnold, London: 271–307.

Robinson J *et al.* (1992) *Policy Issues in Nursing*. Open University Press, Milton Keynes.

Robinson J and Elkan R (1989) *Research for Policy and Policy for Research: a Review of Selected DHSS-funded Nurse Education Research 1975–1986*. Nursing Policy Studies Centre, University of Warwick, Coventry.

Robinson J and Strong P (1987) *Professional Nursing Advice after Griffiths: an Interim Report*. (Nursing Policy Studies 1) Nursing Policy Studies Centre, University of Warwick, Coventry.

Robinson J and Strong P (1989) *Griffiths and the Nurses: A National Survey of CNAs*. (Nursing Policy Studies 4) Nursing Policy Studies Centre, University of Warwick, Coventry.

Robinson J, Gray A and Elkan R (1989) *Griffiths and the Nurses: a National Survey of CNAs* (Nursing Policy Studies 4). Nursing Policy Studies Centre, University of Warwick, Coventry.

Rowbottom S (1978) Afterword. In Kollontai A *Love of Worker Bees*, trans. Porter C. Cassandra Editions, Academy Press Limited, Chicago.

Rogers M (1970) *An Introduction to the Theoretical Basis of Nursing*. Davis, Philadelphia.

Roper N, Logan W W and Tierney A (1983) *The Elements of Nursing*. Churchill Livingstone, Edinburgh.

Roy C (1984) *Introduction to Nursing: an Adaptation Model*, 2nd edn. Prentice Hall, Englewood Cliffs.

Ryan S and Porter S (1993) Men in nursing: a cautionary comparative critique. *Nursing Outlook* 41(6): 262–7.

Salvage J (1985) *The Politics of Nursing*. Heinemann, London.

Salvage J (1997) Changing nursing: changing times. *Nursing Times* 93(5): 24–6.

Shipman M D (1997) *The Limitations of Social Research*. Addison Wesley Longman, Harlow.

Smith I (1975) *Strategies of Social Research: the Methodological Imagination*. Prentice Hall, London.

Smith J P (1987) Report on the 6th International Nursing Conference, RCN Hartlepool Branch, 29 October. *Journal of Advanced Nursing* 13: 303–4.

Smith P and Agard E (1997) Care costs: towards a critical understanding of care. In Brykczyńska G (ed.) *Caring: the Compassion and Wisdom of Nursing*. Edward Arnold, London: 180–204.

Stanley L and Wise S (1993) *Breaking Out: Feminist Consciousness and Feminist Research*, 2nd edn. Routledge & Kegan Paul, London.

Stevens P E (1989) A critical social reconceptualisation of environment in nursing: implications for methodology. *Advances in Nursing Science* 11(4): 56–68.

Stevens P E and Hall J M (1992) Applying critical theories to nursing in communities. *Public Health Nursing* 9(1): 2–9.

Strong P and Robinson J (1988) *New Model Management: Griffiths and the NHS.* (Nursing Policy Studies 3) Nursing Policy Studies Centre, University of Warwick, Coventry.

Strong P and Robinson J (1990) *The NHS under New Management.* Open University Press, Milton Keynes.

Swann C J and Ussher J M (1995) A discourse analytical approach to women's experience of premenstrual syndrome. *Journal of Mental Health* 4: 359–67.

Thompson J L (1985) Practical discourse in nursing: going beyond empiricism and historicism. *Advances in Nursing Science* 7(4): 59–71.

Thompson J L (1987) Critical scholarship: the critique of domination in nursing. *Advances in Nursing Science* 10(1): 27–38.

Tierney A (1990) Strategies for empowerment. *Nursing Standard* 4(47) 15 August: 32–4.

Townsend P and Davidson N (1992) *Inequalities in Health: the Black Report and the Health Divide.* Penguin Books, Harmondsworth.

Traynor M and Rafferty A (1997) *The NHS R&D Context for Nursing Research: a Working Paper.* Centre for Policy in Nursing Research, London.

Turner B S (1987) *Medical Power and Social Knowledge.* Sage, London.

United Kingdom Central Council for Nursing, Midwifery and Health Visiting (1986) *Project 2000: a New Preparation for Practice.* UKCC, London.

Weiss S J (1985) The influence of discourse on collaboration among nurses, physicians and consumers. *Research in Nursing and Health* 8: 49–59.

World Health Organisation (1985) *Targets for Health for All* 2000. WHO, Copenhagen.

Wright S and Shore C (1995) Towards an anthropology of policy: morality, power and the art of government. *Anthropology in Action* 2(2): 27–31.

6

Can nursing research be a caring process?

Gosia Brykczyńska

Nursing research per se is rarely analysed for its ethicacy. It is assumed that research is a good thing, and that nurses should engage in research, understand the research process and implement research findings. This chapter draws attention to some of the more neglected aspects of nursing research: namely, the inherent moral values manifest in the intention to undertake nursing research, the clarity of motivation behind the research process, and the resultant moral obligations on the profession if it wishes to engage in research. Attention is also drawn to the moral significance of the final stages of the research process: the dissemination of research findings and the publication process.

Introduction

There has been much talk recently about the need for an evidence-based practice in nursing. While advocating unsubstantiated nursing practices can be considered at best useless and at worst harmful, the question yet to be answered is: who is to decide on the merit of the 'evidence' cited? Who is to be the arbiter of legitimate practice? Paul Feyeraband, the *enfant terrible* of philosophers of science, rightly noted that over-reliance on research findings can be as harmful as no acknowledgement of scientific endeavour. Indeed, in the introduction to a chapter he wrote in *Science in a Free Society,* he makes the point that because of the blinkered approach that professionals tend to have towards their disciplines, they by default become incompetent practitioners of that discipline. In due course he notes, 'We no longer have incompetent professionals, we have professionalised incompetence' (Feyeraband, 1978, p. 183).

Lest that be said of nurses, there is an urgent need to examine the philosophical orientation of the profession and the type of legitimacy it attributes to nursing research. Some work in this area has already begun (Jameton and Fowler, 1989; Kikuchi and Simmons, 1992) and the purpose of this chapter is to arouse still further, out of a comfortable position, those in the nursing profession who feel there is no need to closely examine the call for an evidence-based practice.

The chapter is presented in four parts. Part 1 addresses the issue of why undertake research in the first place. It looks at the ethical implications of the research intention. Part 2 asks who is the best-suited person to conduct and/or coordinate the nursing research endeavour. The moral responsibilities of the researcher towards patients, colleagues and the health service must be paramount. Part 3 asks whether it is possible, given the potential for conflict of interests, to ever undertake nursing research which is ethical and acceptable to the profession and to the public at large. This section refers the reader to research codes, government recommendations and codes of professional conduct and suggests that while these may be imperfect, they do aim at drawing the researchers' attention to the rights and needs of the public. Finally, Part 4 points out that whereas the greatest emphasis is rightly put on the ethical conduction of research itself – as it is this aspect of the research process that most significantly impinges on third parties and patients – the last part of the research endeavour is also fraught with problems. Increasingly fraud, plagiarism and disreputable research methods are tarnishing the academic, medical and nursing world. This last section looks at the morality of questionable research findings, dissemination and suggests a few ways forward.

Part 1: Why undertake research in the first place?

From the position of too little research activity in the 1950s and 1960s to a current position of 'every nurse a research nurse', the moral arguments have moved from encouraging more research to trying to stem the flood of poor research activity. The same question still needs to be answered: why should we undertake nursing research activities?

One answer to this question has been supplied by the International Council of Nurses (ICN) document to celebrate International Nurses' Day 1996: 'the goal of nursing research is the same in all countries, "To contribute to better health" '. This goal of nursing research assumes, however, that the research will contribute to better health, and that there is a common understanding about the definition of 'health' and of 'research'. The one assumption appears too generous and the latter are definitional nightmares. We could also argue that only a small per cent of nursing research actually sets out to contribute to 'better health'; much of it still reflects the traditional concerns of organization-and-structure and educational issues, although this is beginning to change in favour of clinical research priorities (Marks-Maran, 1994; Rogero-Anaya, Carpintero-Avellaneda and Vila-Blasco, 1994).

In 1987 Nancy Burns and Susan Grove in their popular text book on *The Practice of Nursing Research*, stated that research is necessary and essential for the development of a profession. They stated that it is through research that a scientific body of knowledge is generated and theories are developed and tested, for the purpose of 'planning, predicting and controlling outcomes of nursing practice' (p.4). According to these American nurse–researchers it is the development of the nursing profession that should benefit from research activity. This is very laudable, but can easily be seen to be self-serving: that is, the research can start to serve the purposes and interests of the researchers, which is to have a firmer understanding of the nursing profession rather than of nursing practice. Such research can become in time more and more introverted and self-regarding and nursing researchers can become more and more removed from an analysis of the ordinary practices of nursing, which was their original research intent. Claire Goodman (1989), referring to the history of nursing research and the research practice debate, noted that Dickoff, James and Semradet (1975) reflected that the reason why American nursing research left nursing practice largely untouched was 'because researchers were so concerned with pseudo-technical research methodology that they lost sight of the real problems of nursing' (p.100). In other words, mid-1970s researchers were getting bogged down in research methodology arguments and had forgotten that their focus was to be nursing practice. All academic disciplines and especially practice-based professions have experienced this, and to varying degrees continue to experience this 'problem'. Fortunately, it can be rectified. It is not scholarly attention to research method itself, however, that is concerning some nurses, rather the *preoccupation* with research methodology at the expense of practice issues.

The insistence by health care politicians and nurse leaders for an 'evidence-based practice' in the 1990s only encourages the trite and occasionally superficial response that nursing research is to be undertaken, read and its findings implemented in order to provide nurses with a more rational practice base. This line of thinking assumes, as did the authors of the ICN documents (1996), that the research will not only be of good scholarly quality and practice-related in the first place, but will be read and implemented (Rogero-Anaya, Carpintero-Avellaneda and Vila-Blasco, 1994; Marks-Maran, 1994). Last, arguing for an 'evidence based practice' is not only calling for more clinical research, (and there is no evidence that this is really necessary), but, even more significantly, for a level of discernment and research awareness among nursing practitioners rarely found among most other professional undergraduates and health care practitioners. This in itself is not a reason to abandon the exercise, but as a rationale for more nursing research is rather odd. Either it assumes nursing professionals and students are more mature than other categories of people, or it is imposing a fairly weighty obligation on nurses not imposed on other professions. As Chapman (1991) points out, 'How does a nurse determine which are the appropriate nursing actions for the benefit of the patient?' (p. 29) There are many ways to review courses of actions and many professional decision-making strategies. Hopefully, most of them will be based on logical arguments, rational assessments and an evaluation of the given data. What most research cannot do, however, is, like a television commercial, sell and praise itself. Practising nurses must weigh up for themselves reasons for pursuing particular research evidence on the basis of their own research awareness and personal level of professional maturity, in the presence of conflicting claims and interests. It does not follow necessarily from this, that the profession needs *more* research activity. We could argue that what nurses need to do now, is to read and understand and familiarize themselves with the research that is extant, both in nursing practice and in complementary fields which impinge on nursing.

Finally, the last reason nurses may give for undertaking nursing research falls under the category of personal development and/or academic activity. Nurses often undertake research activities to satisfy university degree requirements, academic institutional policies, employment regulations and, last but not least, sheer curiosity. Some of this research can be useful to the profession and of interest to nursing colleagues, but since this is not the primary reason for the research activity, this is not always the case. It is not surprising therefore that it is often research undertaken for academic purposes that tends to be seen as esoteric or removed from practice – and therefore seen by nursing practitioners as irrelevant to their concerns. Developing various research tools, perfecting questionnaires, looking intently at a particular patient/client population – all such activity is necessary, but unless it is taken further and developed and reintegrated into larger research projects, it is of limited professional use. Returning, however, to the ICN 1996 document, the most important reasons offered about why research should be undertaken, its appreciation promoted and findings implemented are:

1 Research develops knowledge to improve nursing practice for the benefit of patients, clients, families, communities and even nurses themselves.
2 Through nursing research the relevance and effectiveness of established approaches to patient care and health promotion can be evaluated.
3 Research can be focused to demonstrate improvement of health care while containing costs. Nursing research can demonstrate and justify nursing's cost effectiveness.
4 Nursing research can be used to review and strengthen nursing's contribution to society and the health care of society. (ICN, 1996, p. 1)

It is interesting to note that the first and most important reason, according to the authors of this document, is the development of *new* nursing knowledge and insights, which are *practice-focused*, in the interest of patients and clients, communities and discreet population groups. The betterment of nurses themselves is seen as an end product of these activities. Ironically, in this model of nursing research, nurses themselves would have to be seen as clients or potential patients to be the primary focus of nursing research, as would be the case in research on the occupational health of nurses, nurses' work environment, their educational needs, etc.

There is a relatively new movement within nursing ethics that focuses on the concerns of women, and encompasses among other concerns the ethical issues arising from the fact that the majority of nurses are women who are psychologically and socially conditioned to be generous, altruistic and non-demanding (Green, 1982). This traditional gender-based moral position can be seen, however, on occasion, to be detrimental to the individual nurse and thus counter-productive. As Peggy Keen (1991) notes, nurses do not particularly look out for their own welfare, are not necessarily supportive of each other, and yet are urged by nurse theorists and leaders of the profession to be 'more caring'. Keen (1991) suggests that in order to care for others, perhaps we should start by looking more closely at our own needs and certainly learn to be more overtly supportive of each other. Even a quick review of the caring literature will reveal that for all the imperatives that nurses ought to focus more on patients, promote their welfare and protect their integrity, there is no equivalent evidence among this literature, in volume or intensity, which focuses on the nurses' personal integrity and self-preservation needs. Research into these concerns, according to feminist ethicists among others, needs a much higher profile, even if the emphasis seems to be, at first glance, out of alignment with the 'other focused' primary directives of the ICN document. There is certainly some credence to the proposition that we cannot focus on patient needs without some acknowledgement of nursing's own needs.

Parallel to the call for an evidence-based nursing practice is the growing volume of literature by nurses on aspects of caring. Caring is seen as the heart and motivating factor in nursing, where caring, to be effective, is of necessity informed and compassionate (see Brykczyńska, 1992, 1997). Whereas it is easier to see the connection between the need to be 'caring' and for the profession to be 'about' caring – it is somewhat more complex to justify ethical research which will form the basis of informed caring, if the very mechanisms and rationales for evidence-based practice lack moral integrity or a caring ethos.

From a professional perspective, therefore, the many reasons for undertaking nursing research need not of themselves be mutually exclusive or always reflect a conflict of interests, although at different times and for various reasons this might be the case. Most researchers pursue research activities for more than one identifiable reason and focus on research subjects and areas of concern for several reasons – not all of which may be overtly conscious. This reflects the complexity of our approach to this nursing activity (Rogero-Anaya, Carpintero-Avellaaneda and Vila-Blasco, 1994). It needs to be emphasized, however, that the more consciously aware we are of the aims of our actions, the more likely it is that we should be in a position to articulate and prioritize the reasons why we engage in a particular pursuit. Prioritizing and examining various reasons should help ensure that at least some of our identified reasons for undertaking research are not only to serve our own ends, – such as obtain a university degree – but also benefit patients, colleagues and/or the profession.

Nursing research can most certainly help to promote health-focused work, contribute to the decrease in patients' morbidity and possibly demonstrate a reduction in mortality rates. Examples include research in the areas of pressure sores, leg ulcers, breast-cancer awareness, palliative care, perinatal death and post-partem depression. Research effectiveness concerning health promotion, however, is much harder to demonstrate, since this area of work involves so many other extraneous factors, and the time dimensions used for the evaluation of intervention are so much more elastic. There are some areas where it is possible to demonstrate a positive change in people's attitudes and behaviours towards health and health-related issues, such as healthy sexuality, positive attitudes towards breast-feeding, nutrition etc. But even in these areas, it is difficult to state precisely how much of the improvement or change is due to the nursing research activities, and how much they are the result of a general social climate which is ripe for change, because of a concerted multidisciplinary and media approach. To expect nursing research to prove the effectiveness of specific nursing interventions and actions on peoples' health and their associated attitudes, might be rather ambitious. Even determining and defining the nature of beneficial acts towards patients as a result of nursing research can become a complex ethical issue!

Thus, research may demonstrate the long-term damage of heavy smoking on the overall health and well-being of women; but if smoking is considered by the women in the short term to reduce stress and induce pleasure, in the absence of any substitutes, then whatever nursing health-promotion strategy is used to reduce their smoking, an element of paternalism will inevitably be introduced (Macklin, 1982).

Practising the art of nursing, based on research findings, needs therefore to be morally sensitive not only to the reasons for undertaking the research in the first place, and not only to promote what we consider to be in our clients' and patients' interests, but most importantly in a spirit of mature discernment and awe (Marks-Maran, 1994). If the aim of research is to improve practice (wherever that practice may be), then nurses need to take fully on board the moral consequences of their research-based actions. If the current deontological imperative directed at nurses is to base nursing practice on valid and generalizable nursing research findings, then the consequentialist counter-call must be for caution, reflection, consideration of the implications and an appreciation of the action-responsibility (Merrell and Williams, 1994; Holloway and Wheeler, 1995). Only such an approach can ensure a workable moral balance. Ultimately it will be the moral maturity and manifest inherent nursing values that will contribute mostly to maintaining the professional balance (Brykczyńska, 1995). On the one hand we should not be adopting every new finding and revelation without consideration – this can lead to confusion and ultimately cynicism – but nor should we be dismissive of scholarship and sound research. What the medieval philosopher William of Occam stated over 700 years ago still holds true today: *'Entia non sunt multiplicanda prater necessitatem'*: 'Do not multiply your proofs more than is necessary to prove your point'.

Part 2: Who is the best person to conduct and coordinate nursing research?

Assuming that nursing research has a positive role to play in the development and progress of nursing practice, the next major ethical issue to consider is: who should be engaged in research activities? The ICN document suggests that as all nurses are consumers of research, all nurses are involved in research activity, or, as they state, 'all nurses are constantly challenged to review and improve their practice – and thus all nurses have a role in nursing research' (p. 1). From this very broad understanding of research activity to the specific research demands of academic studies, lies a huge grey area of various instances of research activity conducted by nurses with varying degrees of professional competency and research skills.

In the case of the preregistration nursing students, ordinarily there should be little demand for their engagement in discreet research activity, other than laboratory studies, compiling literature reviews and non-person-centred statistical data-processing providing the latter does not violate the 1993 Data Protection Act. The task of the preregistration nursing students (whether or not they are engaged in academic degree or diploma studies) is to learn how to be a nurse: that is, to learn the art, craft and science of nursing practice. Only a small part of nursing practice involves, for some of its qualified practitioners, discreet research activities. Therefore, research appreciation is the primary focus of nursing students at this stage, and an ability to demonstrate the use of research findings.

Post-registration students at diploma and first-degree level pose a totally different problem. Here the would-be researcher is already a qualified nurse (and therefore should already have a basic appreciation of research) but is an unqualified researcher. Curriculum designers need to make clear what are the expected outcomes of their degree/diploma courses with regard to the expected acquisition of research skills. Certainly it is difficult to conceive of an instance where it would be *obligatory* at this basic *academic* level for students to undertake research activities *with* human subjects. The ethical issue raised here concerns the conflict between the lack of research skills by the student and the obligatory respect for patients' right to privacy and non-essential interference by staff and students (Melton, 1992; De

Raeve, 1996). This ethical problem is very similar to the ethical problem of access to patients for educational and clinical purposes by non-qualified staff and/or preregistration students – of all health care professions. In as much as students need to learn their professional skills at some stage with 'real patients', this is overcome by carefully planned educationally sound progressional access to patients, corresponding to the progressional levels of patient morbidity and acuity levels.

Here, however, even the learning encounters are seen as primarily therapeutic interventions. If the students' skills do not match the task required, the nursing activity can and indeed should be performed by a qualified colleague. Supervision is present, and no activity is undertaken that is not within the scope or capabilities of the student. This at least is the accepted ethical compromise as regards an educational scenario. In research activity, however, the levels of difficulty of any particular research project are not always so clear. 'After all,' state some nurses, 'even I can design a questionnaire, conduct an interview, ask questions, measure and assess and evaluate raw data, etc.'

It is not the Mori Poll survey approach of one or two relatively 'public questions' that are the problem here. Should even first-year nursing students go around an entire hospital complex and ask absolutely everyone they meet: 'What do you think of the present government's health care policy?' While within their legal scope to ask the question, it is not addressing the ethical problem. Such a question could be equally well posed by a social science researcher standing at a busy corner of the local shopping mall. No permission would be required in such a case to ask this question and it poses no more than a mild irritation among 'netted' respondents who were too preoccupied or slow to avoid being pounced on. The respondent can always walk away, not answer or display annoyance – or indeed give an elaborate answer. They have the choice to participate or not: after all, the shopping mall is public territory. Anyone can ask questions in public places, and the respondents are there 'on public endeavours'. There is nothing secretive or private about being at a shopping mall. The major ethical issue concerning research in health care facilities is that hospitals are not public places, and patients are seen to be in vulnerable positions. Privacy and protection from abuse of ease of access must be guaranteed, for staff as well as patients (MacNiven, 1993a; Marks-Maran, 1994). Research activities should be undertaken by qualified researchers, and even then only undertaken because the information sought cannot be obtained by any other means, or from any other population group (Kirk, 1990; BPA, 1992; Marks-Maran, 1994). Although not all nurses are in agreement about post-registration undergraduates not conducting small-scale studies, projects and research activities *with human subjects*, the majority of research codes and guidelines about research make a point of stating that research should only be conducted by those qualified to do so (Amnesty International, 1994). It is usually accepted that a minimum qualification necessary to start engaging in research activities with human subjects is the possession of an undergraduate academic degree. Briefly stated, the reason why research activities involving human subjects should be undertaken by those appropriately qualified to do so are:

1 Junior and/or trainee research students are not likely to contribute meaningfully to the profession or patients from these activities, and therefore by involving fellow colleagues and staff, patients and/or clients, violate the basic principle of justice.
2 Junior and/or trainee research students by using fellow colleagues, peers, patients or clients, with little prospect of benefit, risk violating these peoples' sense of security and integrity.
3 Junior and/or trainee research students would find it hard to universalize and justify their actions. Inevitably, there is the heightened risk of depersonalizing the subjects, and using the population group as a means to an end, for example, the completion of an academic programme.

The principle of justice is violated when unqualified persons undertake research with human subjects because, with the diminished likelihood of any professional gains arising from the research, the subjects have been asked to give time and energy to be involved. For example, the distribution of a questionnaire to colleagues and staff may be experienced as frustrating, annoying and a waste of time. Because this activity is a waste of time, it is against a sense of fairness and justice. Since undergraduate students tend to have access to certain designated placements, these areas seem to be unfairly burdened with exposure to small-scale projects. Additionally since there is little natural loyalty to the placement area, little anticipated benefit or positive feedback to the staff or patients is forthcoming at the close of the project. Qualified staff, undergoing continued part-time professional education in the form of an undergraduate degree, may be tempted to undertake a research project at their own place of work. The ICN 1996 document states that: 'Practising nurses who are not trained as researchers make significant contributions to the research process; by their proximity to patients, they facilitate or assist with data collection for nursing and other health-related research projects being undertaken in their work setting.' Rather than set up their own research projects at undergraduate level, it maybe more advantageous to work as research assistants for more senior research nurses. The NHS Management Executive *Health Services Guidelines on Local Research Ethics Committees* makes it clear that one of the points to be considered in regards to ethics in research proposals is the nature of supervision of the research project. Thus 3.2 sub item 5 of Chapter 3 notes: 'Is the investigation adequately supervised and is the supervisor responsible for the project adequately qualified and experienced?' (NHS, 1991 p. 11).

With the steady rise of undergraduate post-registration students, some of whom are keen to undertake research projects in their own work areas, this ethical issue needs to be looked at closely and monitored carefully. Finally, as the NHS (1991) document on LREC's stated: 'There were major concerns about the quality of research' and possibly a need to 'establish a separate research committee to vet the research for quality and the likelihood of its achieving its stated objectives' (p. 7). The increasing problem noted by reviewers of research proposals is their poor quality and less-than-reasonable chance of achieving their stated aims and objectives.

Finally, by allowing undergraduate research students unlimited access to staff and patients, there is the serious danger of obscuring and flooding the work arena. On the one hand staff and patients/clients will find it increasingly difficult to distinguish one research project from another, and thereby disadvantage professional nurse researchers or at least make it more difficult for adequately supervised and competent researchers to gain trust and access to the people required. On the other hand, by too much second- and third-rate research being conducted (not to mention inappropriate research), the clinical areas become overburdened with multiple research projects. On the whole this leads to disillusionment and, in self-defence, can lead to a complete halt to *all* research activity. This is not advantageous to anyone, least of all to well-intentioned, qualified researchers or graduate research students. It should also be pointed out that, increasingly, Trust managers are asking for various items of work-related information in the guise of quality assurance projects, audits, etc. These projects are often inappropriately prepared, conducted and/or their findings under-utilized. The impact on clinical staff is the same, however: an overwhelming feeling of over-utilization of the workplace for the gathering of information, not all of which is strictly necessary or productive and much of which is repetitive (Marks-Maran, 1994).

The second point to consider is the sense of violation of peoples' security and integrity. Staff should not have to feel constantly at the receiving end of critical evaluation or scrutiny. Self-evaluation of a unit is conducted by staff to benefit those self-same staff; student surveys, questionnaires, observation studies, etc. are all conducted primarily to benefit the student. The very role reversal itself, of students looking in critically on staff, is itself unsettling and can be of questionable benefit.

Much as staff may feel their sense of integrity and security is being violated, there is the far greater problem of inappropriate access to patients/clients. One of the basic principles of research involving human subjects concerns the demonstration of proof that the research is necessary and cannot be conducted on or with any other group of people (Amnesty International, 1994). Most undergraduate nursing research (and even some graduate research) is conducted with human subjects in areas where the research is not really vital or strictly necessary. The research study is not likely to add anything new to the existing body of knowledge. Additionally, it is a highly controversial issue among bio-ethicists and the interested public, whether or not it is ethically permissible to simply replicate research studies involving human subjects, for the sake of replication (BPA, 1992; RCN, 1993). With sentient adults it might be possible to gain permission for participation in some form of replication studies, but how would we start to justify a replication study with human research subjects, where the research group were in some way defined as 'vulnerable'? This might be the case with children, frail elderly, psychiatric patients, etc. Certainly the British Paediatrician's Association Ethics of Research Guidelines (1992) suggests that replication studies conducted just for the sake of the exercise should not be undertaken with children. This point is also made by the RCN Guidelines (RCN, 1993).

Either way, the ease of access of *unqualified* researchers, albeit qualified nurses, to patient/client groups leaves us uneasy. It is the ease of access to patients, blurred by the lack of clear distinctions between nursing roles and research roles, that contributes to the problem (Kirk, 1990; Bergum, 1992; De Raeve, 1996). This problem is most acute when nurses undertake qualitative research methods (Ford and Reutter, 1990; Bergum, 1992; Porter, 1993; Holloway and Wheeler, 1995). Especially since so many under-graduate nurses are also part-time students, this blurring of roles when it comes to conducting qualitative research can be even more accentuated (Nolan and Grant, 1993; Holloway and Wheeler, 1995; De Raeve, 1996). Since patients in hospitals and clinics have a right *not* to take part in research studies, and *not* to be approached by would-be researchers, as much as they have a right to participate in studies, this problem is becoming quite important (Merrell and Williams, 1994; Holloway and Wheeler, 1995).

Last, the argument could be used: what if all undergraduate nursing students started to conduct research studies with human subjects? The sheer increase in the volume of work that this would entail for librarians, supervisors, mentors, ethics committees, clinical and academic staff and managers defies description (Neuberger, 1992). There is also the issue of indemnity. Should anything go wrong with the study, or researchers find themselves at the other end of a litigation case, the NHS Management Executive (1991) has made it clear that no compensation is available for cases involving research (Kirk, 1990). Since much of this undergraduate nursing research is neither essential nor therapeutic, there is a growing understanding among qualified nurse researchers and leaders of the pro-fession that it would be far better if research activities with human subjects were conducted by graduate nursing students only, which would auto-matically reduce the number of projects involved and could then be more closely supervised by experienced researchers. As it stands now, by far the majority of academic research is conducted in order to obtain a university academic degree or diploma certificate, and the use of patients/clients and colleagues as research subjects is seen as instrumental in this process. There may be room here for a primary refocusing of the nursing research agenda.

Part 3: Ensuring nursing research is ethical research

If one of the central moral issues in the research debate is the preservation of the personal integrity of the research subject, then the subsequent question that arises must be: how to conduct research in such a way that it is always ethically sound and protects the integrity and dignity of the research subject? Lest we think that there is a form of research activity that does not require ethical scrutiny, such as particular forms of action research, philosophical enquiry, literature reviews, etc, the considered response surely must be that since all our actions are governed by a series of values, and values have moral connotations, no area of our professional work, as no area of our research, is beyond the scope of ethical inquiry (Jameton and Fowler, 1989; Riggs, 1992; Koch, 1995). At its most simplistic level, research is about wonderment and puzzlement, about query, interest and a search for answers – and as the medical philosopher Tristram Engelhardt (1982) observed, 'puzzling about ourselves as much as anything marks us as humans' (p. 75). It is our ability to ponder and reason that contributes so markedly to our humanity, and a major component of our humanity is our status as moral agents.

Common to all research modalities, whether following the scientific–experimental format, or the more subjective qualitative approaches, is the inherent conflict of interests (or potential for conflict) between the researchers' needs and demands and those of research subjects. Mary Warnock (1992), in an extremely readable and lucid presentation of the problem of freedom of choice, notes only too accurately that 'the more another person is seen to have the power to choose, the more *my* power is diminished' (p. 229). By allowing unconditionally for research subjects to turn away from research participation, we allow our own plans to be potentially put aside. The more I try to promote choices for the research subject, the more I run the risk that they will not want to be part of my study! However, it is a central tenet of research ethics that freely given consent must be obtained before enlisting a person as a human subject in a research study.

The process of obtaining consent (otherwise referred to as informed consent) has had a long and fascinating history (Faden and Beauchamp, 1986; Fletcher, 1983). The actual doctrine of informed consent is still being shaped and articulated, but in its broad outline, it bases the need for voluntariness in research subjects and disclosure of information about the project on the two pillars of the theory: namely the Nuremberg Code (1947) and the Declaration of Helsinki (1975). The Nuremberg Code was the first ever articulated medical ethics code specifically relating to the ethics of medical research. It was formulated in the wake of the emerging knowledge about the nature of medical experiments by health care workers of the Third Reich. The vast majority of these experiments were conducted on concentration camp prisoners and members of vulnerable groups, for example the profoundly handicapped, psychiatrically ill, etc. Thus, the first point of the Nuremberg Code is the need for research subjects to volunteer to participate in a study. The Declaration of Helsinki is a further ratification of that code, and it states that 'the interest of the subject must always prevail over the interests of science and society' (Amnesty International, 1994).

If research subjects are to give their free consent to volunteer to be part of research studies, then it also follows that there is an assumption these research subjects understand what is presented to them; the disclosure of information is total; and their freedom to refuse participation in the study will be respected (Silva and Sorrell, 1984; Beck, 1990; Jaggar, 1993). Taken to its extreme position, there is the possibility that very few people would readily volunteer to be research subjects. As Peter Beck (1990) comments, 'Some sort of balance has to be struck between a totally strict, all encompassing regard for the autonomy of an individual patient and such possible utilitarian benefits to allow any medical research to occur' (p. 113).

The sort of balance usually struck is one of mutual benefit, based on a form of moral reciprocity. The health care worker assures safety and continued interest and care and the patient demonstrates altruism in the hope of gaining social and moral approval and respect, if not outright physical benefit – as might be the case in therapeutic research. Alasdair Macintyre (1977), in an interesting early paper demonstrating the inherent moral power of patients (in contrast to the current fashion of proclaiming the unequal powers present between health care workers and patients), notes that rather than be in a subordinate and therefore ineffective position of awe and inferiority, the recognized 'strangeness' inherent within the doctor–patient relationship only serves to heighten the patient's alertness. Thus, 'the very proper fear and suspicion that we have of strangers extends equally, properly to our encounter with physicians' (p. 207). According to Macintyre (1977) patients or clients are leery and mindful of any proposition by physicians; and therefore to state that it is precisely the awe and fear of the health care system that promotes many to volunteer to participate in research studies should be treated with some suspicion. It is not totally clear, however, whether for some patients at least, the power and authority of health care professionals is not indeed the underlying cause why they seem to volunteer so readily to be research subjects. Macintyre, who is well known for his philosophical stance that re-emphasizes the value and worth of personal virtue – ethics – may be assuming a far greater inner resilience and moral awareness among people than is usually present, especially in the context of disease, distress and disability. He rightly suggests that 'nobody can accept the moral authority of another in virtue simply of his professional position. We are thrust back by our social condition into a form of moral autonomy' (p. 210).

The true power and strength of informed consent lies precisely in the possibility that the patient or client has the option of saying 'no' (Meredith, 1993). This power is only authentic, however, if we are truly free morally, socially and culturally to do otherwise: that is, free to choose another course of action (Sim, 1991). Natalie Adams (1977), in an essay looking at the issues of informed consent with prisoners and children, notes in relationship to the significance of other possible options, that in deciding for one option there should always be other realistic options available – especially in the context of therapeutic research. Thus, she notes, 'the kind of situation used as a base is of central importance to the question of whether someone is being presented with a threat or an offer' (p. 116). If the research is presented 'as the only option', this is more of a threat than an offer. True informed consent must always depend on complete optionality and be based on a neutral supposition; even if the denied consent appears to be against the best interest of the would-be research subject (Adams 1977, p. 123).

Some Controlled Randomised Trials (CRTs) prove particularly problematic in this area. The researchers in good faith are trying to prove, beyond sufficient doubt, that therapy options can be genuinely affected: that is, that one treatment modality *is* different (better, worse, totally ineffective, etc), than another. To achieve this, the researchers have to control as many variables as possible, and have to resort to the randomization of research subjects. In non life-threatening situations this research process may be easier to justify and explain to research subjects, but in potentially life-threatening conditions, such as breast cancer, CRTs, whether double-blind or not, can be morally offensive, or at least morally problematic. Some researchers feel that in the context of randomized trials the best ethical option is to conduct double-blind research trials – but these are primarily effective only where medication trials are instituted and could not be employed where more than one treatment modality is proposed. Presumably, radiation therapy could be simulated but it seems a rather awkward and expensive research approach – and, as with all CRTs, it is begging the question about deceit and the non-disclosure of treatment options. Recently, much has been written about the medical, nursing and ethical implications of Tamoxifen trials with women who have had breast cancer or who are most at risk of developing breast cancer (Barnish, 1995). Abuses and mistakes surrounding controlled randomized trials in the emotive and life-threatening areas of cancer care can only polarize patients and health care workers. Recognition that these are emotionally and ethically charged areas should alert nurses and physicians to more openness and honesty, not less, and should prompt nurses to seriously consider their role in such research projects.

Finally, there is the problem of hypothetical versus actual or empirical consent. When a patient, client or healthy person is approached and asked to participate in a research study, this is an instance of seeking for actual consent of a real person, but the research designers had in mind a hypothetical class or category of people who would give hypothetical consent, and in instances of proxy consent the context is effectively necessarily hypothetical. Similarly, when the research proposal went before the research ethics committee, the committee were asked to imagine just such a hypothetical person being asked to participate in this research study, on a hypothetical basis. This point is not, however, just a series of casuistic statements: rather, a reminder, as Alison Jaggar (1993) points out, that when we try to rectify this problem by putting the case for 'perfectly rational fully informed and uncoerced individuals', who inhabit an idealized world, these people bear little resemblance to the rest of us who are 'only partially free, rational and informed – often indeed quite ignorant, damaged, and corrupted – and who inhabit a extremely complex world' (p. 80). The actual problem then appears more true to form if we admit that to gain truly uncoerced informed consent is difficult and possibly in a purist sense unrealisable (Silva and Sorrell, 1984; Dworkin, 1988; BME, 1990; De Raeve, 1996). It is in this context that health care workers often turn to research ethics codes and research committees for help and guidance.

Ethics committees

Before researchers can even start to approach a research subject, their proposal needs to be scrutinized by a Local Research Ethics Committee (LREC). At the beginning of the 1980s, Richard Nicholson, paediatrician and editor of the *Bulletin of Medical Ethics*, undertook a study to investigate the distribution, composition and functioning of LRECs. In his 1986 documentation and analysis of that study, he found much variation and lack of uniformity of objectives among the then-functioning LRECs (Nicholson, 1986). Since that time the Department of Health has not only issued guidelines for the conduction of ethical research but has issued a recommendation that all research involving *patients* must be initially reviewed by an ethics committee (Department of Health, 1991). This recommendation has led not only to an increase in the number of LRECs but also in the volume of work they have had to scrutinize.

The increase in LRECs has led to the realization that there is a lack of uniformity of purpose among the committees; that members of the committees realize a need for research ethics guidelines and a need to inform themselves and health care researchers about the ethical requirements necessary to ensure the ethicacy of research. These realizations and concerns have led in turn to a flurry of ethics of research guidelines, issued by various Royal Colleges, medical establishments, research councils, etc, and government recommendations. The Royal College of Physicians also issued two extremely useful documents about the establishment and composition of LRECs (RCP, 1990) and general points and guidelines concerning research with human subjects (RCP, 1991). These moves were useful and constructive, and if the 1980s were considered the years of growing awareness, concerning the ethicacy of research, the 1990s are the years of implementation of recommendations (Sadler, 1991).

In 1990–91 Rabbi Julia Neuberger undertook to look once more at LRECs to see how they function, after the new guidelines were issued, and to determine their current role, a decade after Nicholson's pioneering survey (Neuberger, 1992). She noted among other things that the composition of the committee membership still varies widely, but that when a nurse was present it tended to make a positive difference. Marianne Rigge (1990) also advocates for more respect to be given to lay members of LRECs. Like Nicholson in 1986, Neuberger was impressed with the impact an articulate nurse can make on the committees discourse and reasonings. Although it is a recommendation of the Department of Health (1991) and RCP guidelines (1990) that a senior practising nurse be part of the standing membership of an ethics committee, not all LRECs actually had a nurse as part of their committee membership, and Rigge (1990) also found that lay representation was sometimes treated very shabbily or under-'utilized'. Meanwhile, the chief aim of LRECs was seen to be the need to review disinterestedly the research proposal assuring the presence of a sound ethical base. This 'sound ethical base' is most likely to be present when the researchers can demonstrate respect for the research subjects, by an openness and a willingness to discuss the research study with them and to dialogue with other health care professionals about issues that arise pertinent to the research question (BPA, 1992; Meredith, 1993). Unless research subjects can really feel free to volunteer to participate or to decline to do so, on the basis of informed consent, it is hard to start discussing the ethics of research; hence the importance attributed to information giving and processing.

Informed consent

Certainly several researchers have commented recently on the problems surrounding informed consent. Dr Nicholson in 1990 edited a collection of recent studies on 'informed consent' in the December issue of the *Bulletin of Medical Ethics* (BME, 1990). Several of the studies reviewed at that time observed in their findings that the language used by researchers to inform patients about research projects was not adequate for the task proposed. The need was seen for the use of plain English, which was not condescending but informative and precise. This was a similar conclusion to the survey done by Silva and Sorrell in 1984. LRECs are supposed to be competent to pick up such failings. When the Department of Health issued its guidelines in 1991, it combined the launch with an emphasis on the Citizen's Charter. The public was to be made more aware of its rights about participation in research, and various interested groups took the opportunity to voice concerns on behalf of others about the research process and participation in studies (CERES, 1990).

All the research studies on LRECs confirm the unease that is present among committee members when research proposals concern minors, vulnerable groups and patients requiring incidental proxy consent (because of temporary incapacity). Much has been written about the problems that arise when research is to be undertaken with vulnerable subjects, who need not just legally binding proxy consent to be given for them, but some personal assent to the participation in the proposed study (Lee, 1991; Alderson, 1993). Gerald Dworkin, a moral philosopher (1988) in a fascinating in-depth study on *The Theory and Practice of Autonomy* notes in Chapter 6 that proxy consent, legal representation and autonomous consent to participate with treatment or in a research study, are not coequal concepts. Whereas it is necessary that someone authorized to do so give consent for therapy as much as for research, proxy consent of an adult is not the same as a child's consent, if that child could consent, for the child at no time 'hands over' their consent. The notion of proxy consent derives from the idea of proxy presence, or proxy votes; it is primarily a sociopolitical not ethical concept. In proxy consent, someone is really making a decision or being present somewhere – on my behalf and instead of me – but mindful of my desires and interests which I have handed over to them. A child or vulnerable adult has interests but these are assumed, and never really 'handed over'; rather, they are benignly usurped. In view of some of these philosophical nuances it is not surprising that professionals working with members of vulnerable groups and undertaking research are increasingly advocating the need to listen to them and respect their assent or refusals. Paediatric nurses, physicians and researchers are well aware of these issues, and most good researchers and clinicians are proud to demonstrate children's assent and consent to participate in therapy and research studies (Alderson, 1990, 1993).

Last, LRECs look at the research design itself. Some of the most difficult research designs to ethically evaluate are clinical trials involving the randomization of patients or studies involving experimental models and multicentre trials (Moran, 1992; Lilford and Jackson, 1995). When a small pilot study was undertaken to look at the 'inter-rater reliability' of different LRECs approach to research proposals, the researchers found that differences of approach do exist. While perhaps inevitable, this is rather disconcerting (Harding and Ummel, 1989).

Nurses' role

The problems addressed up until now appear to have had a medical haze about them. In as much as the bulk of historical scholarship concerning informed consent, therapeutic research and research ethics and research committees in general have been written with a medical rather than nursing readership and bias in mind, this is true (Katz, 1972; BME, 1990). Nonetheless, nurses undertaking research projects however 'trivial' are also bound by the same considerations (Rigge, 1990; Sadler, 1991; RCN, 1993; Parker, 1994; ICN, 1996). In fact, because much of nursing research can be multidisciplinary in nature, encompassing more than just patho-physiological variables and clinical observations but including social, cultural and clinical observations, the opportunities for overlooking ethical considerations and nuances are that much more likely (Marks-Maran, 1994; Parker, 1994). There is also a dangerous myth surrounding nursing research which states that somehow, because nurses care about patients and colleagues, their research cannot do them or their patients harm. This point is also nicely presented in a thought-provoking paper on ethical issues in palliative nursing research (Holloway and Wheeler, 1995: De Raeve, 1996).

Case study

If a nurse sets out to measure the effectiveness of a novel leg ulcer treatment which she has been employing for some time, her research study could easily fall under the heading of audit or quality control. In so far as she is not morally prepared to set up artificially a control group of patients, who would not be treated at all (these would have to be provided by incidental, marginal cases because of self-neglect, misdiagnosis or refusal of treatment) and nor is she prepared to go back to 'old' treatment modalities, her measurement aims are heavily value-laden and prescriptive. She will continue to diagnose and treat according to the 'new' protocol. Her research is simply an internal control and review of this treatment effectiveness as employed by herself and her team. Some nurses would consider this activity only partially falling within the remit of 'research', others would say this sits firmly and comfortably within the nursing research paradigm. What is not clear, is where does the nurse and her 'therapeutic' role begin and end and where does she start to instigate her 'research' role? Where do the two roles overlap and does it make a moral difference? (RCN, 1993; Holloway and Wheeler, 1995; Merrell and Williams, 1994; De Raeve, 1996; ICN, 1996). If the nurse perceives her activities as standard clinical procedure – where evaluation of therapy is an integral part of the treatment design – then she probably would not ask for separate permission of the patients to enrol them into a 'research study' as she does not see her activity as research. Conversely, if she sees this activity sufficiently 'research' biased to account for the need of additional explanation to patients, – she will seek to gain their consent. In many instances the patients themselves may not see, feel or be aware of any extra inconvenience or pressures. It is quite conceivable, however, that because the care and therapy will be closely monitored the patients will need to go to the clinic more often, or for a longer period of time, or have the bandages applied by a specific team who do not speak the patient's language, or are not (initially) familiar with the patient, etc. In other words, however slight from a professional perspective, there is always the possibility of an inconvenience or difference in clinical approach present – and the question remains, depending on the classification of the activity, whether or not a particular moral perspective should be acknowledged, and a research stance undertaken.

Clinical guidelines and codes of conduct

As Dale Beyerstein (1993) acknowledges, there is a strong interrelationship between standard-setting for clinical procedures and codes of conduct. Looking towards codes of conduct and codes designed around ethical issues in research can, however, be frustrating and uninspiring. As Beyerstein (1993) notes, 'Resolving moral dilemmas requires the application of a moral theory which is more general than the moral theory which informs the code of ethics of a particular profession' (p. 417).

When nurses undertake to observe 'influence' or 'guide' fellow nurses in a clinical area, especially in the format of an ethnographic study, or action research, is informed consent required and if so from whom? (Nolan and Grant, 1993; Porter, 1993; Merrell and Williams, 1994; Holloway and Wheeler, 1995). Originally, early ethnographic studies were conducted by anthropologists who took to observing places and societies in cultural contexts sufficiently foreign to the scientist that the 'observer' was the evident 'outsider'. Whether or not permission was sought from the autonomous peoples became somewhat irrelevant to the issue of deceit or covert observation, because it was only too clear for all to see that the observer (participating in the culture or not) was an outsider seeking information, and the local peoples were at liberty to 'include the outsider and cooperate'. The ethics of the research method became much more complicated, however, when social scientists started to use this research modality among cultural groups where they had a reasonable chance of passing unnoticed (Bergum, 1992; MacNiven, 1993a; Merrell and Williams, 1994).

Apart from aspects of deceit and lack of total disclosure, there is the problem of intent (Levine, 1981; Merrell and Williams, 1994; Holloway and

Wheeler, 1995). Research nurses working in a clinical area or with a ...
population, such as drug abusers, may intend to disguise their 'tr...
identity in order to gain more meaningful data. Obviously permission to
work in such a context needs to be obtained (and not just from an ethics
committee), but it is not at all clear from whom – and how much disclosure
would be considered wise and beneficial (Levine, 1981; Macklin, 1982;
CERES, 1990; RCP, 1990; MacNiven, 1993b). In instances like this professionals are likely to turn to their code of conduct, or to their research
ethics code. It is at times like this that the code is put under scrutiny, and
often found wanting. As Beyerstein (1993) points out, the central paradox of
codes consists of the fact that professionals need to think creatively about
their moral obligations and moral priorities, but a code is 'programmed' to
be prescriptive and usually leaves little room for discussion. As Beyerstein
(1993) concludes, 'Being a moral person in society as a whole involves
much more than simply obeying society's laws: it involves paying attention
to moral theory' (p. 423). It is not inconceivable that the moral theory which
guides a nurse researcher to be out of synchrony with the nurses' code of
practice, or as Paul Feyeraband (1981), the philosopher of science noted in a
deliberately provocative essay, 'All ideologies must be seen in perspective
. . . like ethical prescriptions which may be useful rules of thumb but which
are deadly when followed to the letter' (p. 156).

There is another problem inherent in observation and to some extent
participant observation studies: namely, the question of intervention (Merrell and Williams, 1994; Holloway and Wheeler, 1995). At what stage, to
what extent and for what purpose would nurses intervene, should they
observe and be present at a situation that was against standard practice and
deemed unsafe? Any intervention would have to alter, by definition, the
research design and be appropriately 'accounted' for; yet not to intervene
could be clearly seen as against their professional responsibilities and code
of professional conduct. Nurses working within the qualitative research
paradigm would say that this is not a problem for them, as they are present
as researchers who are operating from *within the context* being described,
not looking in from the outside (Merrell and Williams, 1994; Holloway and
Wheeler, 1995). In fact, phenomenological researchers would argue that
since, 'phenomenological research is a human science that strives to "interpret and understand" rather than "observe and explain" ' (Bergum, 1992)
the issue of intervention and even guidance as a possible negative alteration
of the *status quo*, does not arise. Vangie Bergum (1992), working with
pregnant women and new mothers, defines phenomenological research as a
modality that 'explores the humanness of a being in the world'; it is 'a
drama, an *interactive involvement* of both the "researcher" and the "researched" ' (my emphasis). If phenomenological research consists of interactive
involvement with the patient/client/or peer group, then the issue of
'intervention' as it would in an observational study context does not arise.
Here, however, the biggest problem from a moral perspective is the actual

                                                    ...ment of the researchers themselves. That is, more so
                                            ...search paradigm, in phenomenological research the
                                        ...ty of the nurse is under scrutiny and held to account
                                    ...4). As Bergum (1992) observed, 'I, as researcher, cannot
                                ...side the problem I formulate', and indeed she was trying to
                            ...the concept of motherhood, having herself just embarked on
                        ...erience. Sometimes, it is possible to try and 'interpret and
                    ..., as in the process of adjusting to a chronic disease (Morse and
            ...95), or a change or addition to roles, as in Bergum's example of
mo... ood. At other times this might be problematic, not only because of
the nature of the problem under investigation – the process of dying,
undergoing an amputation – but because of the intrinsic 'otherness' and
specialness of the situation (Bassett, 1995; De Raeve, 1996).

Thus, we can empathize with dying patients, as Dr Elizabeth Kubler–
Ross (1969) attempted to do in her now classical study of the experiences of
terminally ill patients in a Chicago Hospital, but she could hardly be said to
have undertaken a phenomenological study of the experience of the dying
moment itself. The moment of death, like the moment of birth, is only
comprehensible to the person who is actively dying or giving birth at that
moment. Qualitative studies have been undertaken with antenatal and
birthing women, but here they can always describe, elaborate and 'fill-in'
the 'emotive' details, in retrospect.

Additionally, as Louise De Raeve (1996) comments, the question must be
posed whether all areas of life (and death is an integral part of life) are open
to research scrutiny, regardless of whether this is classified as quantitative
or qualitative research? It is not labels and methodologies alone that
absolve from moral obligations and considerations; rather, something more
has to be present – possibly a form of reflective wisdom based on moral
development and discernment (Brykczyńska, 1995). As De Raeve (1996)
comments, 'To research at all into the needs and experiences of this client
group could be said to be an affront to the dignity of those people who are
terminally ill and an expression of profound disrespect for the emotional
and physical state of such patients' (p. 24). No amount of justification can
negate the obviousness of this fairly significant observation: it demands
reflection, and research in this area would call for some form of risk–benefit
analysis at the proposal stage which would assure some measure of utility
to the dying patients.

De Raeve cites the early nursing phenomenologist, Jean Benoliel, who in
her 1980 study on research with dying patients justified the nature of her
research work. Benoliel (1980) claimed that it is 'the refinement of knowledge about human responses to dying and behaviours in the context of
life-threatening illness or injury which can only come about through
systematic study of dying as a sociocultural phenomenon' that provides the
moral basis for the research. Part of the sensitivity and moral response of
palliative care nurses must surely be that whatever knowledge they wish to

gain, pertaining to this field of study, it may be more morally appropriate to obtain it via an *ad hoc* and subjective, reflective current and post-fact analysis of events and emotions; rather than via a 'systematic study of dying'. Dying is not just a sociocultural phenomenon; but whatever else we consider it to be, it is also an inexplicable mystery and mystical experience. It is therefore not surprising that many valuable insights in this area are provided by articulate and poetic palliative care workers, rather than researchers.

Finally, De Raeve (1996) cautions against qualitative research nurses, sense of satisfaction and the 'feel good factor' being used too freely as a justification for undertaking studies. Undoubtedly, we often do feel good about the interactions that occur during a study and the sense of completion at the end of research projects can be gratifying. This is especially so when the research study was in an area of moral or social taboo such as birthing or dying. Bergum (1992) pointed out that conducting a qualitative research study with pregnant women, 'brought me back to nursing with reviewed commitment' and prompted questions of health care ethics. Whereas this is a reasonable secondary benefit for the researcher, it would hardly justify undertaking the research study in the first place. How much more relevant are these considerations, therefore, in studies dealing with dying patients? As De Raeve (1996), a palliative nurse herself, concludes: 'Is it justified to make data collection the principal aim and care the sideline, or is one only entitled to research retrospectively having first made care the focus?' (p. 25). These are all problematic areas, with no easy answers.

The more comfortable nurses are in addressing ethical issues on a daily and personal basis, the more easy will become the task of confronting the moral problems inherent and related to the research process. Only a prevailing climate which favours moral priority and an ethic of care will be able to sustain the otherwise potentially dismissive culture of science and research. Science and research need not necessarily oppose a caring, ethical environment – but neither will the research process and a caring nursing modality live comfortably together, without a conscious effort and the personal moral development of individual nurses.

Part 4: The moral significance of research dissemination and implementation

In this last section I wish to raise the moral issues concerning *which* research findings to implement and publish, and *what* to do with scientific and academic fraud and dishonesty. These are areas of the research process that have huge ethical implications but are rarely addressed in the nursing literature, and then only superficially, although this too is beginning to change as nurses are becoming more critical and cautious.

Because of the inordinate pressures put on academic workers to undertake research projects and publish findings in scholarly journals and/or contribute to scholarly works, in order to attract funding, the inevitable problem arises of a glut and backlog of research studies of varying degrees of scholarship, waiting to be published. Many research studies are sufficiently practice-focused that with the recent increase of specialist journals, a good practice-based study should see the light of day, within a calendar year or 18 months of its conclusion, write-up and submission for publication. The peer-review system employed by journals to maintain academic credibility and nursing practice standards may be seen, however, to favour those studies that endorse the *status quo* and comfortable studies that do not 'rock the establishment' over novel and creative approaches, or those that demonstrate negative findings. This is no new phenomena, and much of the writings about change theory and change acceptance, including the scholarly discussions of philosophers of science, address this very issue.

The very acceptance or rejection of a scholarly paper is itself the result of a heavily value-laden judgement process (Marks-Maran, 1994). As Ian Hacking (1981) eloquently points out in his introduction to a collection of papers on scientific revolutions and the history of ideas, we all have an 'image of science', and this image, as likely as not, will be based on the same combination of nine principles. The nine principles which he states shape our vision and understanding of 'science', that is, the nature of research, are realism, demarcation, cumulative knowledge, observation–theory distinction, foundational approaches, deductive thinking, logical precision, context of justification and context of discovery, and finally a fundamental unity (holism) of science (pp. 1–2). This is a very particular list of characteristics that make up in totality or part a particular vision of science, and it is one which is challenged by several notable philosophers of science. The point being made, however, is that wherever we find ourselves on the scientific spectrum and however we view the world, in and around ourselves, we have a more or less conscious criteria for logically approaching and analysing our world. Anyone who presents us with a novel or contrary idea has to either fit their idea into an existing paradigm, demonstrating truth via a coherence theory; or finding no accommodating sub-theory to relate to, even partially, create a new paradigm with new parameters. Obviously, it is far more difficult to do the latter than the former and because of this, even if we have inklings of the need for a 'totally new way of thinking', often the new research-based approach is presented in a format acceptable within existing scientific patterns in order to gain an airing and publication. The ethical problems here are of a particular form of truth distortion, supported by our own, often unconscious reluctance, to endorse the new and 'unrelated'. In nursing practice this may be seen as a reluctance of the established profession (and it is 'established' professionals who act as peer reviewers) to see and consider research findings that support sufficiently novel ideas, which appear to undermine existing practices. Perhaps we do not burn our maverick nurses on the village green, but we do not make their life easy, either (Porter, 1993).

There is also the problem of working in a pioneering area where very few other nurses can legitimately pass judgement on our ideas, scholarly work or research findings. Here, we run the double danger that the person reviewing the paper will either be a friend and/or colleague or possibly even antagonistically inclined. It is very difficult to be objective about the merits of a piece of work if you know the author and possibly have regular professional contact with them. If nothing else, the peer-review system is supposed to be a fair, anonymous appraisal of a colleague's work, not a mutual-adoration society and certainly not an excuse for malice. The second danger is similar to the issue raised already, and concerns the lack of specific knowledge about an area of work to be able to make fair judgement on a submitted paper. This can occur in novel practice-based areas such as assisted conception, where the whole area of work is new and changes are rapid and far-reaching. The danger here is that either the work will be dismissed out of hand, stalled until more evidence to support it is forthcoming, or accepted unconditionally, because of the lack of sufficient expertise to scrutinize the work thoroughly. Obviously all these positions have ethical implications if they play a part in the distribution of research findings and influence the scholarly debates that follow.

Related to this area of concern is the fairly natural problem: that with time, academics and researchers get to know publishers and editors of journals. Whereas this would be considered a 'good and natural thing' in a perfect world, often this can lead to situations where a particular publishing house or journal is favoured over others by researchers and academics, not for sound reasons, but because we are assured a more friendly reception and less critical gaze by one publishing house over another. Editorial boards are not immune to earthly influences, and given the pressures that some academics find themselves under, attempts are sometimes made to manipulate these editorial boards. Usually, it is not overt attempts at controlling publishing house decisions, or influencing editorial consultants of a journal that pose the greatest threat to scholarly integrity; rather, a 'sloppy' morality practised by some academics and practitioners. This is evidenced, for example, by submitting one article to more than one journal at a time, and allowing both to be published, or resubmitting virtually the same work to several journals, and claiming them to be 'original' and separate; and what is always very difficult to prove, utilizing ideas and sometimes even whole papers of students, (plagiarism), and claiming them as our own.

Don MacNiven (1993b), in an interesting essay on academic honesty, highlights the intricacy of complex reasoning that may support such dishonest activities. Usually, the dishonest researcher/practitioner is aware that what they are doing is unethical, at least in some people's opinion.

They justify their actions, however, by a form of relativism and scepticism. MacNiven (1993b) considers these 'intellectual charlatans' as 'pale shadows of the true scholar' (p. 69), and perhaps this is the hidden core of the issue. At any one time, how many true scholars can a society recognize, promote, sustain and encourage to flourish?

Ruby Morrison (1990), in a fascinating general paper on the definitions and detection of disreputable science, addresses all these issues as a nurse, concerned about fraud and misconduct in various areas of scientific and nursing research activities. She notes that 'disreputable science' can occur at various stages of the research process and for various reasons, but many of the practices fall into the category of publishing and dissemination of research findings. Reviewing the literature on the subject, she noted in addition to the issues raised the problems with ghost authorships and irresponsible co-authorships, fragmenting a study unnecessarily to obtain out of it extra publications, and the conduction of trivial studies that would be fairly easy to conduct and write-up. If these latter studies involved human subjects, there is the additional problem of the violation of their integrity. Inevitably the list of 'offences' could continue. The approach of the nursing research community, must be, however, a concerted effort to alter the research climate to such an extent that there is little reason to be fraudulent, and to discourage cheating and actively promote academic honesty (Morrison, 1990).

Fraudulent and disreputable science has been around for many years, yet not everything that appears to be wrong is fraud (which by definition involves malice and forethought). Gerald Dworkin (1983), the moral philosopher, in a paper on 'Fraud in Science', notes that the concept of fraud in science connotes 'the idea of false representation, of passing off as genuine what is only a simulation of the real' (p. 69). Such activity is not done purely by error or happenstance, often it is elaborately planned and exquisitely executed (Levine, 1981; Dworkin, 1983; MacNiven, 1993a, 1993b). The painter who publicly acknowledges that they copy great masterpieces, as an artistic endeavour, is handsomely paid and respected for what must be at the end of the day a formidable talent. This painter is not a 'fraud'. The painter who *secretly* produces frauds, however, and passes them off as 'the real thing' is hardly publicly acknowledged as 'great' for the deceit they perpetrate. Additionally, they are often engaging in criminal activity. Much the same thinking applies to fraud in scientific activities. But as Dworkin (1983) notes, scientists already know all this. Scientists and academicians by virtue of who they are, are concerned with uncovering truth, strive to be original and to have creative approaches to academic puzzles. As Dworkin (1983) states, they 'already accept the moral imperatives against fraud and deception, and accept the virtues of intellectual integrity and honesty' (p. 73). Then why, we may ask, as Morrison (1990) noted, is so much fraud and disreputable scientific behaviour around?

Dworkin (1983) suggests, much as do Morrison (1990) and Ann Clark (1993), that the academic community and professionals must address the problem of why people undertake fraudulent and disreputable scholarly acts and seek to alter the competitive culture that fosters these activities. Dworkin (1983) notes that in the main the 'issues are not moral but political', and Morrison (1990) adds that 'institutions should develop policies which decrease emphasis on quantity of publications and focus on quality ... obviously the more publications, the less time the researcher has to devote to each publication' (p. 912). Clark (1993) also emphasizes that better supervision of students is required. She asks 'whether principal investigations and faculty advisors can provide this level of supervision when numbers under one's guidance are high or when the research is conducted at a remote site.' (p. 116). Clark (1993) states about students what many a nursing colleague might echo, that 'it is disturbing', since 'the behaviours of students may be indicative of future professional performance' (p. 116). It would certainly appear from the cited and reviewed literature that fraud is 'encouraged' among faculty, practitioners and students, where supervision is poor, self-monitoring of institutions a low priority or absent, and there is an all-pervasive presence of a competitive atmosphere.

In conclusion, when fraud is suspected, it should be confronted and quickly dealt with. It is not sufficient to tinker with problems within the scholarly community, without addressing wider and political issues. Nursing research has much to offer patients and the profession but the integrity of research findings is essential if they are to be trusted, disseminated and put into practice. As Clark (1993) notes, 'reasonable dissemination of scholarly work in nursing is critical to the advancement of the discipline' (p. 116). Much is changing, however, and there are legitimate fears that unless nurses themselves monitor their own research activities, the climate will become ripe for abuse and misconduct.

Conclusion

Recently, the British public have been made aware of a major breach of ethical approaches to medical research. In a rare and therefore extraordinary cautionary move, the General Medical Council (GMC) struck off its register a senior GP for failing to conduct medical research in an ethical manner. The deceit perpetrated ranged from non-informing patients that they were part of a medical trial and therefore the non-obtaining of informed consent, to forging research data and claiming to be an 'upright' citizen when he was really dishonest – he was a member of his local ethics committee (*The Times*, 23 March 1996). This form of research dishonesty and fraud *is* rare, but the fact that the GMC decided to remove the practitioner's right to practice is evidence of the seriousness of the offence. It is sad, too, that the practice nurse was also involved in aspects of the deceit.

Nurses increasingly undertake nursing research and are bound by nursing ethical considerations (Marks-Maran, 1994) but they are also increasingly asked and expected to participate in inter-disciplinary research activities or to be research assistants for medical colleagues. In these and every instance, the research activity and the nursing activity *must* be equally ethically sound and compatible. Marks-Maran (1994) in her stimulating review of the ethics of research, observes that 'ethical principles applied to nursing research are the same principles that are applied to nursing practice' (p. 41). To talk therefore of nursing research being a nursing paradox, which questions the moral integrity of nursing research professionals, should be a logical fallacy and an impossibility. That this is not so only reinforces the need for an increase in moral sensitivity, awareness and professional responsibility for all nursing actions, including research activities.

Nurses *do* care about their patients and colleagues, and well-structured, ethically sound research studies can contribute to even better care and professional concern. An admission of nursing culpability and vulnerability, however, would serve to heighten our moral sensitivities, lest they say of nurses as Shakespeare of human weakness, that we are 'Drest in a little authority, Most ignorant of what most assured' (*Measure for Measure*, Act II, Scene 2).

References

Adams N (1977) Medical experimentation: the consent of prisoners and children. In Spiker S F and Engelhardt H T (eds) *op cit*: 111–24.

Alderson P (1990) *Choosing for Children*. Oxford University Press, Oxford.

Alderson P (1993) *Children's Consent to Surgery*. Open University Press, Buckingham/Milton Keynes.

Amnesty International (1994) *Ethical Codes and Declarations Relevant to Health Professions*, 3rd edn. London.

Barnish (1995) Scientific basis, use and nursing implications. *British Journal of Nursing* 4(1): 22, 39–42.

Bassett C (1995) Ethical problems in nursing the terminally ill. *European Journal of Palliative Care* 12(4): 166–8.

Beck P (1990) Informed Consent. In Evans D (ed.) *Why Should We Care?* Macmillan, Basingstoke: 107–15.

Benoliel J G (1980) Research with dying patients. In Davis A J and Krueger J C (eds) *Patient, Nurses, Ethics*. American Journal of Nursing Co, New York.

Bergum V (ed.) (1992) Being a phenomenological research. In *Qualitative Nursing Research* Sage, London: 54–6.

Beyerstein D (1993) The function and limitations of professional codes of ethics. In Winkler E R and Coombs F R (eds) *op cit*: 416–25.

BME (1990) Review: new studies in informed consent. *Bulletin of Medical Ethics* 64: 13–17.

British Paediatrician's Association (BPA) (1992) *Guidelines for the Ethical Conduct of Medical Research Involving Children.* BPA, London.

Brykczyńska G (1992) Caring – a dying art? In Jolley M and Brykczyńska G (eds) *Nursing Care: the Challenge to Change.* Edward Arnold, London: 1–45.

Brykczyńska G (1995) Reflective practice: an analysis of nursing wisdom. In Jolley M and Brykczyńska G (eds) *Nursing: Beyond Tradition and Conflict.* Mosby, London: 9–28.

Brykczyńska G (ed.) (1997) *Caring: the Wisdom and Compassion of Nursing.* Edward Arnold, London.

Burns N and Grove S (1987) *The Practice of Nursing Research: Conduct, Critique and Utilisation.* W B Saunders, Philadelphia.

CERES (Consumer for Ethics in Research) (1990) *Medical Research and You.* CERES, London.

Chapman J (1991) Research – what it is and what it is not. In Perry A and Jolley M *Nursing: A Knowledge Base for Practice.* Edward Arnold, London: 28–51.

Clark A (1993) Responsible dissemination of scholarly work. *Journal of Neuroscience Nursing* 25(2): 113–17.

Department of Health (1991) *Local Research Ethics Committees.* HSG (91) 5, August.

De Raeve L (1996) Ethical issues in palliative nursing research. *Palliative Care*: 22–6.

Dickoff J, James P and Semradet J (1975) Research: a stance for nursing research – tenacity or inquiry? Part 1. *Nursing Research* 24(2) March/April: 84–88.

DPA (1993) *Data Protection Act.* HMSO, London.

Dworkin G (1983) Fraud in science. In Berg K and Tranoy K E (eds) *Research Ethics.* Liss A R, New York: 65–74.

Dworkin G (1988) Consent, representation and proxy consent. In *The Theory and Practice of Autonomy.* Cambridge University Press, Cambridge: 85–99.

Engelhardt T (1982) Reason. In Vaux K (ed.) *Powers that Make us Human.* University of Illinois Press, Urbana: 75–91.

Faden R and Beauchamp T L (1986) *A History and Theory of Informed Consent.* Oxford University Press, Oxford.

Feyeraband Paul (1978) From incompetent professionalism to professionalized incompetence – the rise of a new breed of intellectuals. In *Science in a Free Society.* Verso, London: 183–209.

Feyeraband P (1981) How to defend society against science. In Hacking I (ed.) *Scientific Revolutions.* Oxford University Press, New York, 157–76.

Fletcher J C (1983) The evolution of the ethics of informed consent: In, Berg K and Tranoy K E (eds) *Research Ethics.* Liss A R, New York: 187–228.

Ford J S and Reutter L J (1990) Ethical dilemmas associated with small samples. *Journal of Advanced Nursing* 15: 187–91.

Goodman C (1989) Nursing research: growth and development. In Jolley M and Allan P *Current Issues in Nursing.* Chapman & Hall, London: 95–114.

Green R M (1982) Altruism in health care. In, Shelp E E (ed.) *Beneficence and Health Care.* D Reidel Publishing Co., Dordrecht, Holland: 239–54.

Hacking I (ed.) (1981) *Scientific Revolutions.* Oxford University Press, Oxford.

Harding T and Ummel M (1989) Evaluating the work of ethical review committees: an observation and suggestion. *Journal of Medical Ethics* 15: 191–4.

Holloway I and Wheeler S (1995) Ethical issues in qualitative nursing research. *Nursing Ethics* 2(3): 223–32.

International Council of Nursing (ICN) (1996) *Better Health Through Nursing Research*. ICN, Geneva.

Jaggar A (1993) Taking consent seriously: feminist practical ethics and moral dialogue. In Winkler E R and Coombs F R (eds) *Applied Ethics: A Reader*. Blackwell, Oxford: 69–86.

Jameton A and Fowler M D (1989) Ethical inquiry and the concept of research. *Advances in Nursing Science* 11(3): 11–24.

Katz J (1972) *Experimentation with Human Subjects*. Russell Sage Foundation, New York.

Keen P (1991) Caring for ourselves. In Neil R M and Watts R (eds) *Caring and Nursing: Explorations in Feminist Perspectives*. National League for Nursing, New York City: 173–88.

Kikuchi J and Simmons H (1992) *Philosophic Inquiry in Nursing*. Newbury Park, Ca, Sage Publications.

Kirk E (1990) The nurse and research – legal research. *Nursing Standard* 4(34): 48–9.

Koch T (1995) Interpretative approaches in nursing research: the influence of Husserl and Heidegger. *Journal of Advanced Nursing* 21: 827–36.

Kubler-Ross, E (1969) *On Death and Dying*. Macmillan, New York.

Lee L (1991) Ethical issues related to research involving children. *Journal of Paediatric Oncology Nursing* 8(1): 24–9.

Levine R J (1981) Deception. In *Ethics and Regulation of Clinical Research*. Urban and Schwarzenberg, Baltimore-Munich: 139–54.

Lilford R J and Jackson J (1995) Equipoise and the ethics of randomisation. *Journal of the Royal Society of Medicine*. 88: 552–9.

Macintyre A (1977) Patients as agents. In Spiker S F and Engelhardt H T (eds) *Philosophical Medical Ethics: Its Nature and Significance*. D Reidel Publishing Co, Dordrecht, Holland: 197–212.

Macklin R (1982) *Man, Mind and Morality: The Ethics of Behaviour Control*. Prentice-Hall Inc, Englewood Cliffs, N J.

MacNiven, D (1993a) Experimental ethics. In *Creative Morality*. Routledge, London: 70–87.

MacNiven D (1993b) Academic honesty. In *Creative Morality*. Routledge, London: 53–69.

Marks-Maran, D (1994) Nursing research. In Tschudin V (ed) *Ethics: Education and Research*. Scutari Press, Harrow, Middlesex: 40–7.

Melton G B (1992) Respecting boundaries: minors, privacy and behavioural research. In Stanley B and Sieber J E (eds) *Social Research on Children and Adolescents: Ethical Issues*. Sage Publications, Newbury Park, Ca: 65–85.

Meredith P (1993) Patient participation in decision-making and consent to treatment: the case of general surgery. *Sociology of Health and Illness* 15(3): 315–36.

Merrell J and Williams A (1994) Participation observation and informed consent: relationships and tactical decision-making in nursing research. *Nursing Ethics* 1(3): 163–72.

Moran J (1992) Local Research Ethics Committees: Report on the 2nd National Conference. *Journal of the Royal College of Physicians of London* 26(4): 423–31.

Morrison R (1990) Disreputable science: definition and detection. *Journal of Advanced Nursing* 15: 911–13.

Morse J M and O'Brien B (1995) Preserving self: from victim, to patient, to disabled person. *Journal of Advanced Nursing* 21: 886–96.

Neuberger J (1992) *Ethics and Health Care: The Role of Research Ethics Committees in the United Kingdom*. King's Fund Institute, Research Report 13, King's Fund, London.

NHS Management Executive (1991) *Health Service Guidelines on Local Research Ethics Committees* HSG (91) 5, Department of Health, London.

Nicholson, R (ed.) (1986) *Medical Research with Children: Ethics, Law and Practice*. Oxford University Press, Oxford.

Nolan M and Grant G (1993) Action research and quality of care: a mechanism for agreeing basic values as a precursor to change. *Journal of Advanced Nursing* 18: pp 305–11.

Parker B (1994) Research Ethics Committees. In Tschudin V (ed.) *Ethics: Education and Research*. Scutari Press, Harrow, Middlesex: 72–112.

Porter S (1993) Nursing research conventions: objectivity or obfuscation? *Journal of Advanced Nursing* 18: 137–43.

Rigge M (1990) Who is an expert on ethics? *Nursing Times* 86(11): 22.

Riggs, P J (1992) *Whys and Ways of Science: Introducing Philosophical and Sociological Theories of Science*. Melbourne University Press, Melbourne.

Rogero-Anaya P, Carpintero-Avellaneda J L and Vila-Blasco B (1994) Ethics and research in nursing. *Nursing Ethics* 1(4): 216–23.

Royal College of Nursing (1993) *Ethics Related to Research in Nursing*. RCN, London.

Royal College of Physicians (1990) *Guidelines on the Practice of Ethics Committees in Medical Research Involving Human Subjects*. RCP, London.

Royal College of Physicians (1991) *Research Involving Patients*. RCP, London.

Sadler C (1991) Researching ethics. *Nursing Times* 87(37): 19.

Silva M C and Sorrell J M (1984) Factors influencing comprehension of information for informed consent: ethical implications for nursing research. *International Journal of Nursing Studies* 21(4): 233–40.

Sim J (1991) Nursing research: is there an obligation on subjects to participate? *Journal of Advanced Nursing* 16: 1284–9.

Spiker S F and Engelhardt H T (eds) (1977) *Philosophical Medical Ethics: Its Nature and Significance*. D Reidel Publishing Co, Dordrecht, Holland: 197–212.

Warnock M (1992) *Uses of Philosophy*. Blackwell, Oxford: 223–4.

Further reading

Winkler E R and Coombs FR (eds) (1993) *Applied Ethics: A Reader*. Blackwell, Oxford.

Part 1

Jolley M and Brykczyńska G (eds) (1995) *Nursing: Beyond Tradition and Conflict*. Mosby, London.

Part 2

Gates B (1994) *Advocacy: A Nurse Guide*. Scutari Press, Harrow.
Watson R (1995) *Accountability in Nursing Practice*. Chapman & Hall, London.

Part 3

Beauchamp T and Childress J (1994) *Principles of Bio-Medical Ethics*, 4th edn. Oxford
  University Press, New York.
Edwards S D (1996) *Nursing Ethics: a Principle Based Approach*. Macmillan, Basing-
  stoke.

Part 4

De Raeve L (ed.) (1996) *Nursing Research: An Ethical and Legal Appraisal*. Baillière
  Tindall, London.

7

Researching hidden worlds: dilemmas for nurse researchers

Trudi James and Dawn Whittaker

In this chapter the authors focus on the content and method for researching sensitive topics. They draw on examples from their own research, including the experiences of women undergoing daycare abortion; the perceptions of lesbians and gay men of their health care; the relationship of women nurses and patients in a genito-urinary clinic; and outreach work with women prostitutes. A numbers of issues are raised, such as the ethics surrounding the research of sensitive topics, its emotional impact on participants, the interface with practice, research as a collective process, confidentiality, and the ownership of findings. The authors draw inspiration from feminist research in resolving some of the dilemmas associated with researching hidden, often marginalized worlds.

Introduction

In this chapter we describe and reflect on our experiences as nurses researching hidden worlds. We then explore four key dilemmas that we have both faced doing this work, together with some solutions. Much published research conveys little of the dynamics and difficulties that occur in the active process of designing, conducting, analysing and presenting a study. Research reports are often sanitized and uninspiring, failing to excite and teach us about the dilemmas researchers have faced, and the changes these have brought about for the researcher(s), participants, and the research project as a whole. For us, it is the *how* of research that is the crux of the matter.

Our experience has led us to conclude that the ethical and emotional dimensions of research are often ignored or simplified. In our practice, we have been inspired by feminist research, where the ethical implications of the research relationship, and the researcher's responsibility to protect research participants from emotional harm during the research process and beyond, are central concerns (Oakley, 1981; Kelly, 1988).

There is a tradition in feminist research of attempting to understand and articulate the hidden experiences of women, and other groups of people who are marginalized in our society. This tradition is reflected in the nursing research projects we have undertaken. Trudi has carried out research about women's experiences of daycare abortion, and the perceptions of lesbians and gay men of their health care. Dawn has researched the role of women nurses and the experiences of women patients in a genito-urinary medicine (GUM) clinic, and the occupational health risks and health care experiences of women prostitutes. We should mention that we have been friends for many years, and have also worked together as nurses in a women's hospital. While we have carried out these projects independently, we have been vicariously involved with each other's work, and have supported each other throughout our various research endeavours.

Four research projects

In this section, we each describe the research projects we have undertaken, highlighting the key features and dilemmas of each study.

Research with women having daycare abortions

My (Trudi's) first research project was a study exploring women's experiences of early daycare abortion. I had a dual role as a research nurse, receiving supervision and support from a University Department of Nursing Studies, and as a ward sister, with a clinical commitment in the gynaecology unit where the study was being carried out. I worked as a member of the ward team and attended ward meetings, sisters' meetings and practice-development groups, and participated in teaching programmes for staff. Staff in the unit came to share their concerns, conflicts and problems with me, and I was able to some extent to do the same with them. A rapport developed that I believe would have been impossible to achieve had I remained detached from clinical practice and the day-to-day concerns of the women I was working with and for. I felt strongly that the role of clinical research nurse provided a valuable opportunity to dispel the myth of researchers in nursing living in ivory towers. However, doing research like this as an 'insider' and having a dual research-practice role has its own particular set of dilemmas, to which we return later in this chapter.

I chose a multimethod approach, using interviews, questionnaires, and extracting information from the nursing records. I used these methods with women on the day of their abortion, after discharge at their ten-day nursing follow-up appointment, and (with a small sub-sample) six months later.

The specific aims of my study were to identify women's informational needs, the issues which caused them concern, and their perceptions of what contributed to their emotional well-being. I wanted to reflect and interpret women's experiences of daycare abortion in a way that did not exploit their vulnerability, devalue their experiences, or expose them to pressure or coercion. I also wanted women who took part in the study to know I was cognisant of the inequality that existed between us. I was in a position of authority, while they were in a relatively powerless position. They had to enter a medically constructed, disease-orientated daycare service, and attempt to gain the agreement of two doctors that there were grounds for them to be granted an abortion under one of the four clauses of the 1967 Abortion Act. This was an environment and situation which, I came to believe, was entirely unsuited to meeting what is essentially a social need for well women.

Research with lesbians and gay men about their perceptions of their health care

This is a very personal project that I (Trudi) have been involved in for the last five years. It is an unfunded qualitative research study which is being carried out by a small group of nurses who belong to the Lesbian and Gay Nurses Working Party at the Royal College of Nursing. It is a collaborative enterprise which involves interviews and focus groups with lesbians and gay men about their experiences of nursing care. The origins of the work lay in the worrying reports we were hearing from both lesbian and gay clients and health care professionals, about the inappropriate and sometimes harmful treatment lesbians and gay men were being subjected to in the health care system.We found that while the health care experiences of lesbians and gay men had received some research attention, often in parts of the world that are perceived as 'gay friendly' (for example, San Francisco in the USA), it was a largely unresearched and very sensitive topic here in the UK.

Once again, as in my research with women having abortions, I was aware of the very real power imbalance between myself as the researcher, and the women and men whom I was interviewing. As a team we attempted to address this unequal research relationship, by choosing to use predominantly qualitative methods to gain a more in-depth view of participants' experiences, and by aiming to promote positive changes for them. Where research populations are hidden as a result of their marginalization in society, this power imbalance requires the development of more active strategies than might normally be the case to protect participants from harm. This also extends to the researcher as a participant in the research process.

Research with women nurses and patients in a genito-urinary (GUM) clinic

My (Dawn's) first project was a study exploring the role of women nurses and the experiences of women patients in the GUM clinic where I had worked for two years. Like Trudi, I had a dual role, carrying out the research, and continuing to work as a staff nurse in the clinic.

Strongly influenced by feminist researchers such as Oakley (1981), I began by uncritically accepting the view that I could carry out the research in an equal way that would empower the women participating in the research. Several factors made this position seem a straightforward one to adopt. I wanted to describe and understand the work women nurses were doing in the genito-urinary medicine clinic from their own viewpoint. I myself was one of these nurses. I planned to interview all the nurses who worked in the clinic, and ask a sample of them to keep a diary of their work and interactions with patients. All the nurses were on the same clinical grade as myself, apart from the clinic sister and senior nurse who were on higher grades. They were all interested in and supportive of the project, and appeared to look forward to the opportunity of reflecting on their work. As an insider I assumed they would find it easier to talk freely to me, as they knew I appreciated the difficulties and understood the day-to-day realities of the work.

I aimed to interview a purposive sample of women patients: that is, women who had something they wanted to say about their experiences of using the clinic. I only considered the power relationship between myself and these women in a tangential way, as a concern that their knowing I was a nurse in the clinic would inhibit them from expressing any criticisms they had about their nursing care. I was also very aware that my questions might raise distressing or difficult feelings related to their experience of coming to the clinic (and in particular of having an internal examination), which might not have come to the surface for them otherwise: in short, that the process of the research might harm them in some way. With this in mind, I arranged with the senior health adviser that she would offer support to anyone who needed it as a result of talking to me.

In many ways, the actual process of this project did not highlight to me issues of power between myself and the research participants. I recruited an articulate sample of patients, who told me they welcomed the chance to talk about their experiences both as a therapeutic action for themselves, and in the hope that it would improve things for other women using the service. They also told me they did not feel that they had held back on their criticism or praise. As I interviewed my fellow nurses, I became conscious of their nervousness about this: a fear that they might say something that would reflect them in a negative light, and that I might disapprove of. This was particularly the case for the nurses who had not worked in the clinic for as long as I had. However, all the nurses also told me afterwards that they had enjoyed the process of reflecting on their work.

Research with women prostitutes

My (Dawn's) second research project aimed to evaluate the success of satellite sexual health clinics targeted at women working as prostitutes, and to look more widely at prostitute women's health care experiences and occupational health risks. As in my first project, I had a dual role: working as a nurse in the clinics, and carrying out the research. Two of the main research methods I used were participant observation of outreach and clinic work, and depth interviews with the women.

However, in this second project the issue of my power as researcher in the research process has became more troubling. At the outset of the project, I assumed that because I was known to some of the women and the outreach workers through my work as a nurse in the satellite clinics, they would trust me and realize that I intended to carry out the project in a way that would represent their interests fairly and without sensationalism. In fact, both groups were suspicious of research and its potential to exploit its subjects. The outreach workers expressed concern about the practical and ethical implications of me joining them on their outreach sessions. They were protective of their clients' rights to confidentiality and privacy, and also feared the harm the research might have on their own hard-won access into these women's lives. The prostitute women were suspicious of 'research', and its power to expose or exploit them.

In my fieldnotes my anxieties about the research crystallized around ethical issues: the potential of the research to exploit and betray the women, even to harm them, both in its process and products, and the potential for it alienating women from the clinical services that I was seeking to evaluate and develop.

Four dilemmas for nurse researchers

In this section we describe and explore four key dilemmas we have both encountered in carrying out these research projects: having a dual role as both researcher and nurse; our power and accountability in the research relationship; doing research as an 'insider' – belonging to the group you are studying; and how the feelings of both research participants and research-ers are affected and handled during the research process. We know these dilemmas are faced by many nurse researchers undertaking research on sensitive topics, but relatively little has been written about them in nursing journals and books.

We try to set these dilemmas within the context of the ideas and experiences of those researchers whose work and writing have influenced us and helped us find (sometimes imperfect) ways to resolve them in our research practice. We also flag up key issues for all novice nurse researchers to reflect on, and some recommendations for how they can be supported through the research process.

Dual role: researcher and nurse

Doing fieldwork in your own setting, especially getting started, is nerve-racking. To use a walking analogy, we believe it is common for researchers to make false starts, head off in the wrong direction, find themselves poorly equipped for the sometimes difficult terrain they encounter, and try to do too much and get exhausted and exasperated along the way. However, these are not processes that are usually included in research write-ups – which is a shame, as they can be helpful for novice researchers to read about. Deliberately, then, we would like to talk about the messy nature of getting data on sensitive issues while working in a setting where you already have another role.

Bias

We are both sure that in working as nurses in the clinical areas where we were carrying out our research projects, we influenced the environment and delivery of nursing care in those units. We were also in the privileged position of being able to understand a considerable amount about the ways in which the units functioned: the patterns of communication, the politics of the setting, the formal structures that were in place within the hierarchy, and the not so formal ones.

Rather than viewing this as a weakness, and a potential source of 'bias', we have come to believe it is a strength to openly acknowledge this personal involvement and the ways in which we have used ourselves in both our clinical and research roles.

Certainly having a nursing role facilitated our access into the settings, gave us clinical credibility with nursing and other colleagues and patients, and gave us the knowledge to conduct the research competently and sensitively. However, we also found that the dual research-practice role was fraught with contradictions, and that it created problems and ethical dilemmas for both of us that were stressful and difficult to resolve.

Nurse or researcher?

Like other nurse researchers, we have found a key ethical dilemma is the conflict that can occur between our role as researcher and our clinical role (Field, 1991; Lipson, 1991). These roles can become highly intertwined, but remain conceptually different. Central ethical issues are those of intervention and advocacy: what should we as nurse researchers do in situations where our professional values tell us to intervene or advocate for a person, but where research values are also in operation?

On several occasions, we have both decided to abandon our research values. For example, in the daycare abortion study, Trudi chose to care for a woman during her hospital stay and sit with her during her abortion (which was carried out under local anaesthetic), after this woman had confided in her about the sexual violence she had experienced and expressly asked for her support. Here, as in other situations, the therapeutic imperative to support this woman as a patient overrode the research imperative. So rather than continuing to recruit other women to the study from that morning's admissions or attempt to use this woman's experiences as 'interesting' data, it felt the caring and right decision was to honour her request.

Whilst we have learnt that it is vital to set boundaries and be aware of own limitations, we believe that research-mindedness should not take precedence over empathy and a desire to respond to another human being in distress and in need of our professional help. We do not think it possible or advisable to attempt to suspend or separate the centrality of caring that is part of our being nurses, from ourselves as researchers. If we acknowledge and include our caring orientation in our research endeavours, it offers us the potential to develop these skills concurrently. We can do this in ways that minimize the sense of unease and insecurity that come from trying to disassociate from our feelings and knowledge base – for both ourselves and those affected by our research. We suggest ways of managing this feat later in the chapter.

But we also offer a word of warning here. As Gosia Brykczyńska states in Chapter 6, just because nurses have a caring role does not mean that their research will not cause their patients or themselves harm. She asks where do the research and therapeutic roles overlap, and does it make a moral difference? Many skills which nurses learn are conducive to enhancing the rapport and trust which yield better data in research, such as interviewing, listening, and the intentional use of self (see Lipson, 1991). One of the moral issues becomes purporting to use these skills for one purpose, while actually using them for another. The ambiguity in roles can be a source of discomfort, particularly when there are few or no avenues of support available to those who conduct and take part in research.

Maintaining role clarity

We have both found that our patient research participants merged the nurse and research roles, and often cast us in our more familiar nursing role, with all its attendant expectations.

For example, Dawn found that the prostitute women found it easier to accept her in her role as the clinic nurse. This situation was exacerbated by using the unobtrusive method of participant observation, where there were no instruments like tape-recorders or questionnaires to signal that this was research. It was also hard to raise the research aspect of what she was doing on hectic outreach sessions and in busy clinics, where contact with women could be very brief, and they were often absorbed and preoccupied by their work or health situation at the time. In these circumstances, informed consent to the research became a very grey area.

We are both sure that some of our patient research participants did not have a chance to understand and consent to the research component of what we were doing. Even if they had, there was also the issue of whether we were trading on our nurse roles to encourage women to give us information that we would use for the research. An illustration of this, which we have both experienced, is when a woman has revealed a past history of sexual abuse to us in a research interview, prompted by our knowledge about other related and intimate aspects of her life which had been revealed to us in a clinical situation. This blurring of roles also has implications for informed consent. If patients are primarily viewing the researcher as a nurse, they may feel obliged to reveal the kind of personal information they would not normally share with other people, and which they would have withheld if the researcher role had remained dominant for them.

A similar situation exists with nursing and other colleagues. We have both found that although colleagues were first wary of our research role and our power to judge and evaluate their professional behaviour, this role was quickly subsumed to one of team member as we worked alongside them. It then became problematic as to how informed their consent was to the research in our informal interactions with them, and also in how we represented them in our writing.

The transition from nurse to researcher is not a straightforward one for colleagues to adapt to or understand. Trudi's fieldnotes describe the shock of her first days of data collection:

> I thought that by simply changing my clothes – swapping the sister's uniform for my own clothes and burying my name badge deep in my pocket – I would go unnoticed by staff and patients alike and merge into the background. However, quite the reverse has happened: I appear to be even more noticeable. Doctors are infuriated when sister won't sort out a problem, and think I am just being obstructive and unhelpful. When other nurses know that I am on the unit I'm often consulted about clinical issues and have ended up acting as a cover for meal breaks. (If this means I'm the difference between them getting a break or not then there's no choice to make.) While patients keep asking me to walk with them to the toilet or check their pads. It must be the way I behave, how others respond to me and I to them. I radiate 'nurseness' even when I just walk through the unit. How can I change this – to be one thing one day and another the next?

This extract also illustrates how we have found it hard personally to differentiate the two roles of nurse and researcher, often finding ourselves in a limbo world between the two. In Dawn's research with prostitute women, her fieldnotes are peppered with references to the pull and conflict between the roles:

> I think a problem is this 'in-between' position I find myself in – not one thing (a nurse) or the other (a researcher). I feel like I'm not doing either. Now all my questions and concerns have an ulterior motive – and I both want to know, and to protect the women from telling me too much.

In these projects, we have frequently found it easier to present ourselves as nurses and not researchers, and become swept up in clinical activity and commitments. Other nurse researchers, such as Nicky James (1984), have also described the powerful pull toward adopting an active nursing role. This tallies with Janice Morse's wry observation:

> I find that nurses are the worst people to send in to do participant observation because they cannot sit in the corner and 'do nothing' . . . before you can turn around they are working! (Morse, 1991)

Adopting a nurse role is sometimes unavoidable. However, we have only learned slowly how to steer a course between our resolve to collect the data, and the need to respond to emergencies or the requirement for an extra pair of hands.

Preparation and support

Our experience has taught us that not only do nurse researchers need to make their role functions and priorities clear to patients and colleagues, they also need to think through and be clear about them to themselves. Translating and integrating roles is actually very hard for first-time researchers. Preparation is vital. While it is difficult to anticipate the exact nature of events that can happen during a project, it is helpful to think in advance of fieldwork what likely conflicts of interest may arise and how you would handle these if they occurred. We believe that it is essential for novice nurse researchers to have close supervision and support in order to carry out research that is rigorous and ethical, and which successfully negotiates the problems of having a dual role.

Power in the research relationship

Who are you to do this?

It may seem unremarkable that the community or group being researched rarely have a say in the choice of researcher, and the subject or mode of enquiry. Yet as researchers exploring hidden worlds we need to consider questions, such as: Would this particular group of people, given a choice, want to expose their lives to us? What do they stand to gain or lose by permitting us to enter into their lives? We should always ask how our 'right to know' is balanced against participants' rights to privacy, dignity and self-determination.

These questions are especially pertinent where individuals or groups manifest what have been labelled 'deviant' lifestyles or behaviours, as was the case in all the research projects we have undertaken. How could our research participants know that we would accord them respect, be non-judgemental, and take care in how we represented them in the world? After all, researchers are not usually engaged in their studies solely on the basis of altruism – our goals are generally more utilitarian and self-interested. We have found it is helpful to bear in mind the following questions, 'Why are you asking those questions?' and 'Do you really need to know that?' It is naïve to think that as researchers we can walk into a situation and start asking questions about sex and death, for example, and not consider the effects these may have.

Our accountability to those we research is rarely made explicit. Ethical codes of conduct for nursing research often comprise lists of practical procedures or steps to be followed which do not deal in any depth with the complexities of the research process. For example in Chapter 6, Gosia Brykczyńska raises the issue of 'vulnerable' groups. Ethical codes of conduct and research guidelines generally allude to the responsibility of the researcher to protect vulnerable individuals or groups. These are usually taken to be children, or more recently the elderly and mentally ill. However, the issue of what constitutes a 'vulnerable' group is a complex one. Lesbians and gay men are vulnerable as a result of their marginalization and stigmatization as a group; prostitutes for some of the same reasons. We need to consider how we can best practically protect those who are made vulnerable by society throughout the research process and afterwards, not just prior to obtaining ethical approval. Critical self-appraisal should be ongoing in order to discern and reflect on our own values and moral judgements where they may be proscriptive or hurtful.

Feminist researchers have long struggled with these complexities, and the issues of power and control in the research process. A concern for the ethical implications of research relationships is a basic principle of feminist research (Wise, 1987). Here we consider two elements of the research process central to both the feminist debates about research ethics and our own experiences of doing research: rapport and reciprocity, and the representation of research participants and researchers in published accounts.

Rapport and reciprocity

At the end of the 1970s, feminist researchers argued that the orthodox methods of social research exploited and objectified women as research subjects. Feminist researchers were urged to create an egalitarian research process characterized by authenticity, mutual self-revelation and reciprocity.

These themes of reciprocity and rapport were famously taken up by Ann Oakley (1981) who proposed a model of feminist interviewing based on her own experience of interviewing women. The research relationship, she argued, should be founded on a genuine rather than an instrumental rapport. As the researcher, Oakley demonstrated reciprocity in the relationship through answering questions in the interview, and offering social support through and beyond the research. She found that she came to be regarded as 'a friend not purely a data gatherer'.

Like many other feminist researchers we were strongly influenced by this model research relationship, and attempted to adopt it as a matter of principle. For example, Trudi offered emotional support to women under-going daycare abortion, as she encouraged them to reflect on their feelings about the experience. In her fieldnotes she wrote:

> Sharing their feelings about an experience that has often been regarded as something shameful to be hidden, and making suggestions about how the care could be improved, did enable a sense of reciprocity to develop between us. I was very aware they were allowing me entry into a hidden world I could not gain a deeper understanding of without their help. Almost all of the women involved told me they felt it was a way of giving something back to the nursing staff who they felt were caring and supportive, which might in turn help other women in the future.

Another way Trudi chose to empower the women participating in this project was to ask them at each stage if they wished to withdraw from the study and, if not, how they were feeling about continuing. This strategy has been called 'process consenting' (Munhall, 1988). We both believe it is the researcher's responsibility to gain consent not just at the inception of a study, but throughout the process. This is because you can never anticipate what may happen in the life of a project: situations, feelings, dynamics change.

However, as other feminist researchers have realized in the years since Ann Oakley wrote her seminal paper, we have learned that the process of doing research remains an unequal endeavour, and that the power relation-ship between us as researchers and our research participants needs to be acknowledged and dealt with. It is dangerous to assume that because we are women keen to research other women's lives with sensitivity, care and respect that this is enough to protect them from harm. 'Women' are not a simple or unitary category, and real barriers are created between us by class, race, age, culture and sexuality. Feminist researchers tend to be from more powerful groups than the women (and men) we are researching. Indeed, following the 'friendship' model of research relationship can raise expectations and induce dependencies in research participants. Ultimately all that they confide in us becomes grist for the research mill, and we are far freer to leave the relationship. Although some feminist researchers view it as part of their feminist commitment to become involved in the lives of the women they are researching (Cannon, 1989), others have asked: 'With how many dozens of people can a researcher, however sincere, however femin-ist, consistently communicate?' (Patai, 1991).

Representation and the politics of interpretation

As nurse researchers we are in the privileged position of studying others' experiences and lives. Yet whether or not, or indeed how, those who choose to be part of our research efforts have any say in the research process, in the interpretation of the data, or in the generation of knowledge about them-selves is often an absent element in published work. This is an ethical issue that should be of great concern to those of us doing research with vulnerable groups, as our power to represent them can add to the inequities they face in society. For example, researchers have indicated that there is considerable homophobia and ethnocentrism in nursing, and a denial of the care needs of culturally and politically marginalized groups. It is our responsibility to ensure that we do not impose further harm through the research process and its products (a principle often referred to as non-maleficence).

We have been greatly concerned in our projects that we could harm already vulnerable research participants in the way we represented them in our research reports. We believe that the issue of how data is used is also an ethical matter. We were both acutely aware that in our respective studies we had the power to bring into a more public arena the experiences and voices of women and men from disenfranchized groups. While this seemed a valuable opportunity there was also the risk that it might mean making them more vulnerable to attack both physically and morally – a double-edged sword. Hidden worlds by their very nature provoke curiosity. When representing the views or experiences of those from counter-cultures, great care is required that they are not made public in ways which may promulgate voyeurism and contribute to damaging stereotypes. For example, the current fascination for and interest in women who sell sex and the lives of lesbians has frequently been manipulated by the media, who have tended to sensationalize rather than sensitively reveal the issues about these communities.

This extract from Dawn's research diary serves to illustrate some of the dilemmas we have encountered in representing our research participants:

> As I approached the prostitute women about interviewing them in depth about their health and working lives, I learned that many of them had been exploited by researchers in the past. From their accounts, it appeared that many of these 'researchers' were journalists, whom they had talked to 'in confidence' – only to find their stories (and in some cases, photographs) splashed all over the papers. When I asked women if they would talk to me, I was careful to explain how I would ensure their confidentiality and anonymity (for example, through removing any identifying information from tapes and transcripts, which would be stored securely; and presenting what they said in ways that would not identify them individually), that this project was supported by the health service, and aimed to investigate ways their health and safety at work could be improved. However, even with the women whom I had come to know well (and who were confident and articulate about their work with me, and the clinic and outreach workers), and whom I felt sure would agree – I met with polite refusals.
>
> I became highly sensitized to the fact that prostitution was a sensational as well as a sensitive topic. This was a hidden, misunderstood and stigmatized world, which was constantly exposed to the prurient gaze of the public, mainly through the media. It was represented in ways these women found hurtful, objectifying and dangerous to themselves. Anonymity and confidentiality were

real, live concerns – many women told me they lived in fear of being exposed to their partners, their families, and the law.

   Their response forced me to face up to my own position. How much could I honestly say I was doing the project 'for them', and how much was I doing it for my personal and academic self-interest? This was combined with real anxieties about the kind of observational data I was collecting, and how I was going to analyse and present them in a way that would not just excite the prurient curiosity of an academic and possibly wider audience, and serve merely to expose the women to more harm. They would be harmed if I added a romanticized or dramatized gloss to the stereotypes of what the lives of prostitute women were like, but detailed descriptions might also expose them to more tangible harm from punters, police, and their landlords and pimps (if they had them). Writing this, I can see that I may have had, and still have, delusions of omnipotence, but these fears about my power in the research process have begun to overwhelm me.

If we choose as researchers to act purely as ciphers in order to be 'true to the data', this can constitute an act of betrayal. Yet is it right to deselect research data in anticipation of harm? This crisis of representation has been an enduring concern for us in our work with vulnerable groups, how what participants tell us gets out into the world. We can illustrate this with an example from Trudi's lesbian and gay research project. When she interviewed lesbian women with current or past mental health problems, they were cautious when it came to discussing issues of self-harm with her for fear of how this might be interpreted by a wider audience. The worry for these women and the research team was that self-harm would be interpreted as indicative of the general mental instability of lesbians. To counter this interpretation, the research team sought to locate these women's experience within the social and cultural inequalities that bound them, such as the historical construction by society of lesbianism as pathological.

   Another strategy we both adopted to mediate our power to represent others' lives and experiences was to check back with those we researched that we had written an honest account of what they had told us, and that our interpretations would not, in their view, cause them harm, individually or as a group. This was also a way of acknowledging that we the researchers did not have sole ownership of the data.

   However, we are also aware that these now established strategies are open to criticism. For example, Sue Wise (1987) is scathing about strategies for democratizing the research process. She argues with cogency that there is no one collective interest for research participants from oppressed groups; that researchers cannot control how their findings are used; that incorporating a structural account invalidates participants' experiences as 'false consciousness'; and that:

> To offer research subjects 'the right to reply', and to call that 'protecting their interests' is fundamentally dishonest ... because we know they won't do it and, if they do, who will take notice? (Wise, 1987)

Feminist researchers have increasingly recognized the complexities of representation in their work. Over recent years, alongside a continuing commitment not to objectify research participants in the research process, there has been a move toward researchers taking responsibility for interpretation of the data they collect. The ethical principle is translated into one of rigorously connecting experience to understanding, and through making the process of data production and interpretation clear.

This principle has also been extended to making the researcher(s) visible both in the process and products of research projects. We would argue strongly for self-reflectivity in the research process. Reflecting on our own identities, and why and how we have come to choose a particular sensitive subject area, has been helpful when examining the impact our motivations and beliefs have had on the design and conduct of our studies. How you come to be known by those who consent to take part in your research can strongly influence the outcomes of the study. Differences and conflicts are part of everyday life but are rarely paid much attention in research reports, as they seem to be regarded as an indication of defective planning. Belgrave and Smith (1995) provide an honest account of these ethical and epistemological (the way in which knowledge is generated) concerns in their collaborative, interpretive study of Hurricane Andrew in Florida. In doing so they explore the impact of their different theoretical perspectives, personal experiences of the event and their gender on the ensuing analysis and production of their findings. Making ourselves visible in research reports will make for more truthful representations of the process of doing this kind of work, which after all is about forming relationships, with grantholders, other researchers, participants, the data we generate, and the people with whom we share our findings. It is incongruous to reflect only one side of those relationships.

Insider or outsider?

Many nurses choose to research subjects they have some personal knowledge of within a particular hospital or community setting they are familiar with. It is not unusual to find that within a short space of time they are experiencing conflicts of interest. Some of these we have already mentioned in the section on dual roles. Others are more particular to being an identified, or hidden, member of the group you are researching.

Trudi's account of her collaborative research project about lesbian women's and gay men's experiences of health care shows how being an insider can have an altogether different meaning:

As a lesbian, I share identity with the group of people I am researching. This has had the advantage of facilitating access to a hidden population with a particular cultural identity that I have an intimate understanding of. Lesbians and gay men I have interviewed often state that they are tired of having to play an educating role when they are ill and in need of informed care. A typical

comment is: 'I should be coming out to teach them, but when
like hell, you know, educating people is the last thing you want

My status as an insider means I can use my 'bias' as a way of en
to feel comfortable to talk to me about the issues that concern then
there are problems associated with what ethnographers call 'going i
perhaps more appropriately for me, being native.

The researcher as vulnerable

Lee (1993) talks of stigma contagion, of the detrimental effects of con
out as part of a group that are perceived in a negative light by mainstre.
society. Trudi writes about this experience in relation to her research wit
lesbians and gay men:

> As part of a team of researchers involved in this project who are open about
> our sexual orientation, we have all felt vulnerable at times. Dealing with
> homophobic comments and attitudes, having to change our telephone num-
> bers as a result of lewd and threatening phone calls, and the reactions of some
> colleagues who have been observed to physically shrink from us in corridors,
> are not imaginary occurrences. Career prospects can be jeopardized, and while
> we are all employed full-time in other capacities – researching the care needs of
> lesbians and gay men is not a priority for funding bodies – exhaustion easily
> sets in. There has been tremendous resistance and a reluctance to accept the
> idea that research of this kind is warranted.
>
> Feelings of great frustration and disappointment have affected us personally,
> as we are confronted with the stories of women and men who have found
> themselves helpless in a health care system that has on numerous occasions
> pathologized their lifestyles, denied them equal access to care and treated them
> with contempt. We have often been deeply affected particularly by the stories
> of those caught up in the mental health system who have survived in spite of,
> rather than because of, their treatment.
>
> As a team of researchers we have found coping with the feelings that
> researching sensitive issues engenders to be central to the process of ethical
> decision-making. It is our view that there needs to be more value placed on
> intergroup dynamics in collaborative working – time for the discussion of
> personal ethics and room for the emotional distress that can be created for both
> researcher and participant in listening to and recalling disturbing personal
> accounts.

Privilege and inequalities in 'insider' research

The following extract from Trudi's research diary is an attempt to highlight
some of the ethical dilemmas surrounding the status of nurse researcher as
being in a privileged position while being bound by the structural and
societal inequalities consequent on belonging to a stigmatized group:

> I was contacted by a young woman who had been sectioned under the Mental
> Health Act and sent to a secure unit 150 miles away from her home town,

because of the lack of psychiatric beds and suitably trained staff in her area. She contacted me via a friend. She was aware of our research project, and urgently wanted to be interviewed by one of our team. Her friend indicated that she was terrified the patients and staff of the secure unit would discover she was a lesbian, and that she would be both psychologically and physically at risk. As a team of researchers we should have gained clearance through the local ethics committee to interview this woman. However, the concerns expressed by her indicated that she would have been made even more vulnerable and at risk of harm had we exposed her by following standard ethical guidelines to apply to the local ethics committee in order to speak to her. I decided to visit her as a 'friend' and interviewed her secretly. The experience was nerve-racking, but left me in no doubt that fearing the consequences of revealing one's sexual orientation, while feeling trapped within the mental health system, does not augur well for the recovery of emotional well-being.

After the interview, it was vital that I was able to turn to other members of the research team to talk about the responsibility I felt to do something to help, and my feelings of powerlessness in being able to change much, if anything, for her. Identifying as another lesbian with her in this situation, what were the boundaries of my role? I had felt discomfort about acting like a spy in the unit, and unease about being covert to the unit staff about my intentions in visiting her. Of course, apart from a dangerous gut reaction to smuggle her out in my car, I could not single-handedly combat the structural and interpersonal homophobia she was experiencing.

The need to work out our boundaries as researchers is often something that has to be decided on the spot. Inappropriate spontaneous reactions grounded in over-identification can result in harm to both ourselves and those we research. Alternatively, to comfort ourselves that we too are members of an oppressed group, while retreating to the 'comfortable heights of the academy' (Patai, 1991) will not make the world a better place for those we leave behind. To do this takes energy, commitment and political activism – and means taking risks.

While we are aware that Trudi's choice of actions in conducting the interview secretly could be criticized, we have chosen to bring this particular experience out into the open as an example of an ethical dilemma for nurses who do research in hidden worlds.

The structure and organization of the health service and the care delivered by individuals within it has been found to be heterosexist in nature (Stevens, 1995). While health care professionals and the institutions they serve remain homophobic, lesbians and gay men will continue to be seen as 'the other', marginalized, isolated and silenced. Ethically, in order to honour the need to protect research participants from harm, it is our belief that those who are vulnerable in this way should be allowed to speak without fear of recrimination. Indeed, it could be argued that this is a civil right.

Managing feelings

Feelings of research participants

Before setting out on our own research projects, we were aware of other researchers' accounts of how sensitive research had profoundly affected the feelings of those involved in it. For example, Sue Cannon (1989), who interviewed women who were dying of breast cancer, described their experience of the research process as 'lengthy and emotionally demanding'. She found that most women cried at some time during the series of interviews she conducted with them, and she often had to halt interviews temporarily as participants became so distressed. Liz Kelly (1988), who studied women's experiences of sexual violence, realized that many women were 'very shaken' during or after the interview. The interviews awoke buried memories of incidents of sexual violence for some of the women, which they disclosed to her for the first time.

As we have already discussed in our accounts of our work, we were both concerned about the emotional impact of the research on our research participants. We feared it would be too intrusive, and cause them to reflect more than they would otherwise have chosen to on their feelings about personal and difficult experiences.

On several occasions these fears were born out, as is illustrated in this account from Dawn's research diary of her relationship with one of the prostitute women who agreed to be interviewed in depth:

> As she talked about her life and the work, Barbara became progressively more emotional and upset. As the interview progressed, she started to reveal some very personal information to me. One of these disclosures was that she had been sexually abused as a child, and that she repeatedly re-enacted this scene with clients who wanted her to act out their abusive fantasies with them. We were both visibly affected as she talked about this. I asked her if this upset her, and she told me it always brought back her own memories, and that afterwards she had to 'sit and console herself'. However, she saw this part of her work as a way of preventing other girls going though the trauma she had suffered.
>
> After the interview, Barbara wanted to talk to me several times at the clinic, and told me more intimate things about her life, asking me for my advice and help, and often crying inconsolably.

Managing research participants' feelings

We both took steps to try to minimize the potential distress our projects could cause research participants, in both the design and conduct of our studies.

The following is just one example of this from Trudi's daycare abortion study:

> I was familiar with research that had shown that women regarded consultations with health professionals as hurdles to overcome in the race to get an

abortion. There was evidence that women did not share their worries and concerns with staff for fear of being denied an abortion. Many women do not expect health care professionals to hold positive views and feelings about abortion. This is not unrealistic as nursing staff have been found to have strong and negative attitudes to women undergoing abortions. Why then should women regard me as a nurse researcher in any different a light?

Decisions about the timing of my research interviews encapsulated these issues and also involved ethical dilemmas. My own experience as a gynaecology nurse led me to believe that women were unlikely to want to discuss their feelings with me at their first outpatient's appointment. I had observed the range of protective strategies women adopted to shield themselves from negative attitudes at this time, combined with their uncertainty about access to an abortion. I felt that they might view an interview with me as part of the medical process of assessing their suitability for abortion. In addition, it would have meant substantially extending what was already a lengthy process, which involved seeing a doctor, phlebotomist, radiologist and nurse counsellor. If women had made a choice not to tell others in their lives, or had children to collect from nursery or school, or had work commitments, this could only have added to their anxieties. Even though it would have been a fruitful source of data for me, I therefore chose not to approach women at this time when they were likely to be emotionally vulnerable, and where I may have caused distress and harm.

Trudi was surprised to find that many women who participated in this study found the experience positively beneficial. They told her that it helped them to feel part of a shared experience, and they saw it as an indication of concern for their needs, as a way of conveying understanding and support and of reducing their isolation. This tallies with the experience of other researchers who found that participants often appeared to gain some therapeutic benefit from being involved in research. Patai (1991) concludes that the opportunity to talk about one's life is 'an intrinsically valuable experience'.

However, there remains the possibility for poor or inappropriate management of participants' feelings in the research situation, and this potential is acute when using the method of qualitative interviewing, which we chose to use in all these projects. Often, as indicated in the account of Dawn's interview with Barbara, interviews can seem to turn into counselling sessions as difficult feelings are aroused in participants.

We are both of the opinion that the research interview is not a counselling session, not least because research participants have different motivations for agreeing to participate. Research participants are not only, if at all, seeking to achieve a greater sense of well-being. But as interviewers, we often use counselling skills, and inevitably some of the same psychodynamic processes come into play when one person asks another to talk about personal experiences, which may bring up painful memories and feelings, perhaps previously never shared. It is not surprising, therefore, that respondents look to the person asking these questions to provide them with support, information or advice (Batchelor and Briggs, 1994). We believe that it is an ethical imperative that the researcher address the needs and expectations raised during the research process, and recognize the painful feelings which may have been aroused. This may mean enduring the pain with participants during the interview itself, and establishing referral sources if the process has raised issues which they wish to resolve.

However, we believe that it is not necessary or desirable for us as researchers to feel we have to meet all these needs ourselves. In all these projects we sought to establish referral sources, where immediate therapeutic intervention or long-term support was available for research participants if difficult issues and feelings had been triggered for them by our research instruments.

But these strategies did not always work in practice. Here is the continuing extract from Dawn's fieldnotes about her interview and subsequent contact with Barbara:

> I was so affected by what she told me that I was unable to support her. The interview fizzled out without me checking out her emotional state, although she told me as she left she did not know who she could talk to about these things. There is no doubt that some of what she said really shook me up. Afterwards I felt very emotional myself. It feels really hard about what I should do with all this stuff. There is the issue of my support, and support for the women I talk to – and how I should process and present what they say.
>
> I am extremely unsure of my boundaries in these situations. I have told her that I can talk to her during clinic time, but that I am not a counsellor. If she wants I can refer her for some counselling support with the clinic health advisers. But she said she did not want this.

Researcher support

In describing the dilemmas we have experienced, we hope it has become clear that the process of researching sensitive topics has often been distressing for us as researchers as well as for our research participants. Doing research can be a lonely and painful process, and in all these projects we have been glad of the emotional support of friends and colleagues. Indeed sometimes we have been dependent on this support in maintaining our own mental health, and in enabling us to continue with our projects.

Ensuring that researchers are appropriately supported during the research process is also an ethical issue. This is particularly important for novice researchers, who have no experience of the feelings research can arouse, and for fieldworkers who are working alone. Preparation for the potential emotional impact of research and the anticipation of ethical dilemmas are a key element in this. We have found that our experience in dealing with emotionally charged situations as nurses does not necessarily translate into the research context, and we feel that this kind of preparation is especially relevant for nurses carrying out research in familiar settings, with the role conflicts and culture shock this can bring.

Like other researchers we have found the support systems that existed for us have been *ad hoc* and informal. We would like to make the case here for the establishment of more formalized researcher support, based on the model of supervision which exists for counsellors. This would involve regular meetings with an independent, trained supervisor to discuss how the research is affecting and being affected by the researcher's feelings. Dawn was fortunate in arranging this kind of formal supervision for herself in her research with prostitute women, when the feelings this project was arousing in her threatened to overwhelm her. She writes:

> Supervision has helped me to incorporate practical ethics into the project, provided me with emotional support, and enabled me to focus on and explore the feelings the research has aroused in me.

The suggestion of the need for a structure of therapeutic support for fieldworkers is not new (Lipson, 1991; Batchelor and Briggs, 1994). But we suggest that a formal system of supervision has clear benefits for the integration of ethics and feelings into the research process.

Conclusion

As researchers, while we may focus on what and how our respondents think and feel, it is our own thoughts, feelings and values which shape how we interpret and represent them. As we expose the former to scrutiny, so we should the latter. We hope these reflections on the 'how' of the research process will be useful to other nurses with an interest or involvement in researching sensitive topics; and that we as nurse researchers can begin to integrate these issues into our research practice, and not just express the ethical and emotional difficulties of research in conversations with other researchers, or tuck them away into the appendices of research reports. It is not just through the end results of research that we gain knowledge, but in the creative process of doing it. Research is a social endeavour, and we should incorporate its emotional dimensions and the opportunity it gives us to develop greater ethical integrity in the conduct of our work.

References

Batchelor J and Briggs C (1994) Subject, project or self? Thoughts on ethical dilemmas for social and medical researchers. *Social Science and Medicine* 39(7): 649–54.

Belgrave L L and Smith K J (1995) Negotiated validity in collaborative ethnography. *Qualitative Inquiry* 1(1): 69–86.

Cannon S (1989) Social research in stressful settings: difficulties for the sociologist studying the treatment of breast cancer. *Sociology of Health and Illness* 11(1): 62–77.

Field P A (1991) Doing fieldwork in your own culture. In Morse, J (ed.) *Qualitative Nursing Research: a Contemporary Dialogue*. Sage, London.

James N (1984) A postscript to nursing. In Bell C and Roberts H (eds) *Social Researching: Politics, Problems and Practice*. Routledge & Kegan Paul, London.

Kelly L (1988) *Researching Sexual Violence*. Polity Press, Cambridge.

Lee R M (1993) *Doing Research on Sensitive Topics*. Sage, London.

Lipson J (1991) The use of the self in ethnographic research. In Morse J (ed.) *Qualitative Nursing Research: a Contemporary Dialogue*. Sage, London.

Morse J (ed.) (1991) *Qualitative Nursing Research: a Contemporary Dialogue*. Sage, London.

Munhall P (1988) Ethical considerations in qualitative research. *Western Journal of Nursing Research* 10(2): 150–62.

Oakley A (1981) Interviewing women: a contradiction in terms? In Oakley A(1993) *Essays on Women, Medicine and Health*. Edinburgh University Press, Edinburgh.

Patai D (1991) US academics and Third World women: is ethical research possible? In Berger G S and Patai D (eds) *Women's Words: the Feminist Practice of Oral History*. Routledge, New York.

Stevens P E (1995) Structural and interpersonal impact of heterosexual assumptions on lesbian health care clients. *Nursing Research* 44(1): 25–30.

Wise S (1987) A framework for discussing ethical issues in feminist research: a review of the literature. *Studies in Sexual Politics* 19: 47–88.

Further reading

Nielson, J McCarl (ed.) (1990) *Feminist Research Methods: Exemplary Readings in the Social Sciences*. Westview Press Inc., London.

Reinharz S (1992) *Feminist Methods in Social Research*. Oxford University Press, Oxford.

Renzetti C M and Lee R M (eds) (1993) *Researching Sensitive Topics*. Sage, London.

Skeggs B (1994) Situating the product of feminist ethnography. In Maynard M and Purvis J (eds) *Researching Women's Lives from a Feminist Perspective*. Taylor & Francis, London.

Titchen A and Binnie A (1993) Research partnerships: collaborative action reseach in nursing. *Journal of Advanced Nursing* 31(1): 1–12.

8

Reflections on a bordercrossing: from ward sister to clinical nurse specialist

Helen Mann

This chapter is about transition and reflection on new roles. The author uses systematic reflections on 20 years as a ward sister to describe the shift towards her new role as a clinical nurse specialist. The author describes the process of documenting her skills and transition within a changing health service using a research approach to practice. The chapter is written as a narrative in which a number of important issues are highlighted: the ward sister as culture bearer and team leader; her sources of power and control over staff and territory; the setting of frameworks and standards which shape the nature of nursing on her ward; the relationship between intuition and knowledge; and an analysis of how nurses undertake emotional labour and how it relates to positive and negative attitudes towards patients.

Introduction

The creation of this chapter began when I left my ward sister's role of 20 years. I wanted to capture something of the uniqueness of that role before I embarked on something new. In discussion with a friend, a research nurse and former colleague, we spent a day tape-recording my memories and reflections. In other words, we used a research approach to document some of the unique skills of being a ward sister. Later I found myself not only reflecting on my ward sister's role but also documenting the transition to a new role within the context of a changing health service. I was describing a bordercrossing from a general to a specialist role and some of the obstacles I encountered.

I have written the chapter as a narrative account in a discursive, experiential way. I wanted to do this before referring to the literature on the various topics which eventually emerged. In the context of research agendas I have framed my chapter in the spirit of inductive enquiry, starting from my frontline experience and seeking the formal theories later.

If clinical nurses are going to influence the setting of nursing research agendas, it is important that they describe their hands-on experiences in order to make them visible. But often they don't have the opportunity to do this. In my own case, it was a struggle for me to write this chapter for a number of reasons. My clinical workload was emotionally and physically demanding so that when I came off-duty, the last thing I wanted to do was write about what I had just left behind. Furthermore, I was often too exhausted to put pen to paper. But I did it, determined to give voice to what nursing on the frontline is all about. I also found that in the new look health service I could use this same voice for working with managers to negotiate better conditions of patient care.

The letter

When I was planning this chapter the following letter came to my attention. What makes it surprising is that it was written about a ward in a hospital with a reputation for excellent nursing care. The letter demonstrates that in this ward things had gone badly wrong. In particular the values and culture generated effected not only how the patient and her relatives felt but also her recovery. The patient was admitted for the management of advanced cancer and although it was clear her condition was terminal, her family believed that had she continued to receive such poor care on the ward her death would have been hastened.

> Our mother was admitted to your hospital via the Accident and Emergency Department and from there transferred to Bennett Ward. She gradually improved after receiving blood transfusions and intravenous fluids and a week after admission the decision was made to drain her abdominal ascites.
>
> To relieve the discomfort from the tube and from the draining itself she was started on morphine elixir. Her condition began to get worse, she was now not able to feed herself or drink without help. She became disorientated and confused.
>
> Our family's opinion was that a combination of medication and not being able to feed herself was contributing to this deterioration in our mother's mental condition and general health. However, discussions with the nursing staff, either when we visited the ward, or by telephone always resulted in defensive comments about the care she was receiving, and there was very little concern for her general well-being or how her relatives were feeling. When we expressed our worries, or made suggestions, the response from the nurses was very negative.
>
> Meanwhile, our mother's condition continued to worsen. She had developed pressure sores over her heels and sacrum, her urine output was low and concentrated and she was too confused and shaky to be able to drink as much as she needed.
>
> Fortunately, at this stage, our mother was transferred to a local hospital where she made a remarkable recovery. In a caring and loving environment her condition slowly improved and now she can participate in conversations, and feed herself.

We feel that this improvement is due solely to the quality of care she is now being given. Nothing else is different. When she was with you, it would appear that no one acted on her behalf; that little attention was paid to her right to be treated as a human being with feelings. Nor was her family, when they expressed their anxieties and worries, treated with respect or understanding.

I was haunted by such statements as 'In a caring and loving environment her [confused and dependent] condition slowly improved and now she can participate in conversations and feed herself' and 'We feel that this improvement is due solely to the quality of care she is now being given. Nothing else is different'. I returned to these statements again and again and they provoked me to ask a number of questions: What are the factors which make the quality of nursing care on one ward different from another? How are decisions made about what is considered to be important? What are the influences which contribute to the predominant attitudes and skills on a ward? What part do different members of staff, and most importantly the ward sister or charge nurse, play in creating the atmosphere in which patients are nursed and formulating a philosophy that governs their care. I aim to address these and other questions throughout this chapter.

My trajectory

My reflections on and subequent narrative about my nursing trajectory have grown out of my transition from being a ward sister to becoming a clinical nurse specialist for the care of stroke patients. For nearly 20 years I had managed acute medical wards. In the four years leading up to my role change, I was the ward sister on an 18-bedded medical ward and stroke rehabilitation unit. Patients were transferred to this 18-bedded unit from all over the hospital to facilitate their discharge home. They stayed for periods ranging from three weeks to three months. The nurses worked closely with a multidisciplinary team comprising a physiotherapist, occupational therapist, speech and language therapist, social worker and a neurologist. Even though I had been an experienced ward sister when I first began working with the team, I felt myself to be a more able and complete nurse four years later. This was because I developed new skills which meant I was better at managing stroke patients' problems with mobility and communication. I also learnt to recognize their special needs. The difference between regaining self-esteem and making progress or not, was dependent upon them being nursed by staff who allowed them to practise the skills taught them by the therapists. Within the acute part of the ward, we sometimes nursed patients with newly diagnosed strokes which allowed us under my leadership to build up our expertise even further as a skilled nursing team in the care of stroke patients.

Despite our successes, the ward was grossly underestablished and dependent on pre-Project 2000 students or agency staff to make up the full staffing complement. In order to improve continuity I designated an F grade and an E grade staff nurse to be team leaders. Diligent attention to the off-duty rota, and careful planning of the skill mix, allowed the two team leaders to spend a minimum amount of time on night duty so that they could share their skills and knowledge during the periods of most activity on the ward. I would divide my time between the teams, filling the gaps and ensuring I spent enough time nursing those patients whom I judged warrented expert nursing intervention.

Although I ensured that both the stroke and acute medical patients on the ward received the same high standards of care, I was aware that patients with strokes, especially those whose lives had changed so much as a result of their disabilities, would benefit from more information and explanation. I was keen to specialize and use the experience I already had to focus on this patient group, whose needs were so little understood. During my last year on the ward, events facilitated my transition to a specialist role and the creation of my new post as a clinical nurse specialist for the care of stroke patients.

Changes in the health service, the creation of a purchaser/provider divide, increased attention on the consumer voice and the 1992 publication of the *Health of the Nation* targets, all played a part. First, the results of a project set up by the purchasing health authority to investigate the needs of people with stroke and their carers, were published. Stroke had already been recognized in 1992 as one of the *Health of the Nation* targets (DoH, 1992):

> Approximately 12 per cent of all deaths in 1991 resulted from stroke which is also a major cause of disability, particularly amongst elderly people. Stroke accounts for 6 per cent of total NHS expenditure and results in the loss of about 7.7 million working days each year.

Following the Health Authority report, discussion groups and a multi-disciplinary conference were organized. From these initiatives evolved the final recommendations for improving stroke services within the Health Authority. They included the establishment of a designated area within the main hospital for the admission, treatment and nursing of acute stroke patients.

Around the same time that these activities were taking place, there was a major reduction of the medical beds within the hospital as part of the general austerity measures being taken in the health service to cut costs. The floor on which I worked was subsequently closed and my ward disestablished. The rehabilitation unit was relocated and the acute medical beds incorporated into a larger ward elsewhere. The nursing team was split up and reassigned to work in these areas. These changes were associated with great sadness and uncertainty among the staff.

On the positive side, however, the establishment of a 28-bedded general medical ward which was much closer to the therapy departments allowed the hospital management to carry out the purchaser's requirements for creating an acute stroke unit. Although the unit would only have eight beds and therefore only cater for a proportion of the total number of patients admitted to the hospital with stroke, the plan was to admit them for a stay of up to four weeks. Within that time it was expected they would either be discharged home, transferred to the rehabilitation unit or to the ward of their admitting medical consultant. This policy would reduce the number of times these patients were moved around the hospital. Since my experience was that each adaptation a patient made to a new nursing team involved some functional loss, it was hoped that by keeping their movement within the hospital to a minimum, it would be possible to reduce their length of stay.

As the newly established clinical nurse specialist I planned to spend part of my week on both the acute and rehabilitation stroke units and to see as many patients with stroke in the rest of the hospital as I could. My post was hospital-based but I saw myself as a resource for community nurses who might seek advice for patients being transferred home.

I thought out what I considered to be the main components of my role: clinical judgement, innovating and creating, empowering and enabling, striving for excellence, practising accountability and autonomy and being an educator, change agent and support for nurses, carers and patients. My role would also involve health promotion and helping patients to cope with the restrictions that handicap imposes. The job description I developed with my nurse manager (The Director of Medical Nursing) included elements that I knew to be my strengths: being an identifiable expert in the care of stroke patients by setting clinical standards of care by role modelling; liaising with the hospital bed manager to ensure that stroke patients were nursed in the most appropriate area; and facilitating discharge and adequate follow-up.

The hospital's Director of Nursing Services (DNS) had been instrumental in helping me to create this post. She had seized the opportunity that arose from bed closures to establish a post for which I had identified a need. In turn my recommendations were in line with hospital, health authority and government policy for improving the prevention and treatment of strokes.

The DNS and I both felt that my experience and skills made me ably qualified for my new role. I had credibility as an expert in stroke care with nursing, medical and therapy staff; particular communication skills both in enabling and empowering nurses and patients; and past successes in managing change.

I was excited and enthusiatic about my new role and looking forward to this next step to bettering the care of stroke patients. It did not feel as if I was moving away from my skills as a ward sister but moving towards a new interpretation of my nursing skills.

Reflections on a trajectory

So what have reflections on my trajectory to do with setting nursing research agendas? First, I do not think I could have used systematic, analytical reflections without some basic research skills which I acquired on the ENB's Research Appreciation course, No. 870. This course gave me an understanding of basic research techniques, how to formulate research questions and to make links between clinical practice and research findings. Charting one's trajectory, which is popular among ethnographers, helps to examine the interface between the personal and the political; the micro and the macro; the individual and the organizational. By seeing my transition from ward sister to clinical nurse specialist in the context of wider organizational and political change, I was able to meet my personal needs as well as make a contribution to the development of nursing and patient care. I also showed how it was possible to take control of situations rather than be controlled by them. I was not prepared, however, for some of the difficulties I experienced when my new role clashed with nursing values and cultures which were different to mine. Although emotionally demanding, the conflicts I experienced gave way to new insights and understandings about the nature of nursing to inform practice, education and research. I also saw the importance of taking the initiative rather than being overtaken by events. The chapter is organized into sections around nine themes which emerged from writing about my experiences of transition from ward sister to clinical nurse specialist.

The ward sister's management style, emotional labour and the effects on patients

During 20 years as a ward sister I had developed a problem-solving and reflective approach towards patient care. It was important for me to seek a rational explanation for why things happened and for what we did. It was also important to identify and validate the complex components of nursing and to acknowledge that our work was not always straightforward. The ever-changing priorities of an acute medical ward impose time constraints and mean that nurses have to make choices and delegate. Honest explanations rather than defensiveness seemed to me to be an easier way of accounting for nursing actions, or omissions, to patients, relatives and colleagues.

This philosophy necessitated exploring patients' feelings about their illnesses and hospitalization. We needed to make sense of their attitudes and actions. What nurses interpret as 'unreasonable' behaviour in patients can often be ascribed to either a lack of information and explanation or concern that their viewpoint is being overlooked. A key element of nursing practice is to be able to understand what a health problem, or disability means to a person (McMahon, 1991) and one of the most important of nursing roles is to give patients relevant information about their condition and treatment, and ways of coping with both (Wilson–Barnett, 1986).

Every ward has its own distinctive management style and the leadership style of the sister dictates what the priorities are (Smith, 1992). A series of research studies have demonstrated the critical role of the ward sister in setting the tone and standards for patient care (Pembrey, 1980), controlling the general atmosphere of the ward, and being the key to its success (Ogier, 1982; Fretwell, 1982).

One of the students interviewed by Smith (1992) described every ward move as a 'culture shock'. Each ward operates in its own way. Pembrey (1980) describes the patient and their relative as 'vulnerable' and 'so dependant on the ability of the ward sister to ensure that he is properly nursed'. Lewis (1990) observes that the overwhelming evidence is that for good or bad, the tone of the ward and the care within it is dependant on the personal philosophy of the ward sister.

My personal philosophy was shaped in part by role models I had been exposed to as a student nurse who even in the early 1970s organized their wards around patient allocation and listened to nurses' evaluations of their care at the end of each shift. They had a very clear idea of what the role of the nurse was, and defined what nursing was within their wards. The ward sister in her role as supporter of her staff, and architect of nursing work and organization, sets the emotional tone of the ward (Smith, 1992). It is the sister who decides how much attention is to be paid to the staff's and the patients' feelings, and what the reward systems should be. Work organizations are sites where individuals make meanings for themselves and have their meanings shaped (Fineman, 1993). The ward sisters' sense of values shapes what staff members see as gratifying in their work and defines those aspects that they are prepared to work hard at.

In planning care I taught nurses to include the patients' perspectives as well as the staff's, to try and avoid being judgemental, ascribing feelings to patients or projecting their own feelings on to them. We had to learn to identify the separate nature of these two strands, and to manage them both; not consider them one and the same. Since the main planners of care are trained nurses and they can be the ones who spend the least time in direct contact with patients, it was vital to discuss care within a forum where qualified and unqualified staff came together. This was invariably the shift handover. Within a setting in which what nurses had to contribute was considered more important than their ranking within the nursing hierarchy, we could examine both patients' and nurses' emotions.

'Nurses need to be cared for and to be recognised as individuals within their own right' (Kirkpatrick, 1967). Despite an awareness of how it should be, Smith (1992) still found that students were incredulous at the lack of support they got from their teachers and ward sisters. If my philosophy, which placed the patient at the centre of the ward and its activities, was to be practised, then caring for the nurses was vital. They needed to feel valued and know that their feelings about work and patients could be expressed, accepted and seen as valid. They needed to feel free to explain their rationale for their behaviour towards patients. The views of every member of staff had to be acknowledged as important, if they were going to give credence to their patients' views and allow that to influence how they cared for them. I also had to acknowledge what hard work giving credence to patients' views was. The non-physical, non-technological side of nursing makes considerable demands on staff. Being patient, listening and showing concern, taking on the anxieties of both patients and carers, not to mention the anxieties of other nurses and other disciplines, takes up energy and increases stress levels.

This emotional or sentimental work or labour that is carried out in the hospital setting, is recognized as being necessary, time-consuming and difficult (Smith, 1992, Strauss *et al.* 1982). The nurse has to manage both her own and the patient's emotions, and yet appear calm, and sustain in patients the sense of being looked after. Emotional labour is work that is invariably invisible and often unacknowledged.

Being honest about how patients made us feel rather than judgemental about their behaviour made it easier to admit intolerance or dislike for some of them. I would teach nurses that there was no reason why they should feel compelled to like all of a group of some 20 disparate people, but that they did need to recognize that all patients had a right to equal standards of care. Separating out the nurses' feelings from the patients' needs made that care easier to give.

Our goals with awkward, unlovable, or disruptive characters was to get them through as quickly as possible. Because they seemed unlikely to contribute in any positive way to the work of the ward (Johnson and Webb, 1995) careful evaluation and clarity in planning their goals was essential. Motivation and rewards for the nurses when dealing with these patients had to be clearly defined: permission to be proactive and creative in managing them; praise and acknowledgement of the nurses' efforts and successes; reflection on the skills learned in the course of the exercise; increased confidence in their ability to manage a similar situation in the future; and the satisfaction of successfully meeting a difficult challenge.

Giving care in a consistently non-judgemental way meant, however, that we were more likely to be able to influence a patient's behaviour (Stockwell, 1984). Not stereotyping them allowed them space and opportunity in which to modify their behaviour without losing face. We were not defining how we thought they might act in the future, and so not depriving them of opportunities to change. In being given no history, they had no grudges or scores to settle.

Nurses feel guilty about labelling patients and so creating an atmosphere where it was not legitimized or rewarded, made for more honest discussion and increased support for each other. Johnson and Webb (1995) observed that when nurses carry out high quality care and interpersonal interactions with patients whom they perceive not to be liked, they have to do it more or less covertly in order for their dissidence not to become evident to the dominant members of staff. It takes time to do, and circumstances and patients are often such that it is unavoidable. It can be demanding and immensely tiring, yet on many wards emotion work is not valued or recognized as part of nursing. Smith (1992) observed that nurses who felt appreciated and supported emotionally by the ward sister had both a role model for emotionally explicit patient care, and felt able to care for patients in a similiar way.

As the above account demonstrates I had clearly acquired a variety of skills and experience during my 20 years as a ward sister. I was keen therefore to integrate and develop them in my new role as a clinical nurse specialist. I drew on the relevant literature to assist the process.

The clinical nurse specialist role

Since the 1970s, the clinical nurse specialist (CNS) role, which originated in North America, has become well established in Britain.

Boucher and Bruce (1972) defined the CNS as a skilled practitioner, competent researcher, knowledgeable change agent and accomplished educator. Twelve activities which were seen as an essential part of the role were listed by Aradine and Denyes (1972) and similar key factors were identified by Castledine (1982). These included being involved in direct care, and being responsible and accountable for nursing actions; being an expert in the nursing process approach to care and coordinating care with other professional health workers; acting as a consultant to others and educating both health care workers and patients; liaising between hospital and community; involvement in clinical nursing research; and freedom and flexibility within the role. The UKCC (1994) envisages advanced nursing practitioners as being pioneers developing new roles.

Specialization is seen as allowing nurses to refine their practice by narrowing the range and increasing the depth of their knowledge and skills (Castledine, 1995). Yet they need to keep the central dimension of their role as consistently pertaining to direct clinical practice (Wilson–Barnett, 1995). Castledine (1995) saw the needs that drive the nurse specialist as including that to 'explore new knowledge about the nature of nursing and to satisfy the curiosity of the committed, intelligent, creative and sensitive nurse'. He also saw the role as a response to the demand of the public for more expert nursing care. Wilson–Barnett (1995) recognizes the expansion of specialist nurses in recent years as, in part, arising from patient need. In chronic conditions, such as stroke or those that are under-treated or under-recognized, non-specialists confess to inadequate skills and knowledge. Smith (1990) examines Holt's (1984) work on the development of the role and the suggestion of a sequential pattern of development. The strongest component is seen as that of clinical practitioner, with the aspects of role model, teacher, researcher and change agent strengthening over time and with growing confidence.

Sequential pattern of development (Holt, 1984):

1 Increasing confidence in the knowledge and theoretical applications of the nursing speciality through direct care to individual patients.
2 Planning with others for care of groups of specialized patients.
3 Gradually increasing the sphere of influence in working with nursing colleagues and staff, to change the nursing care of patients within the specialization.
4 Developing small clinical research projects and sharing the results with nurses and other disciplines.
5 Planning with others for changes in delivery of care based on experience and research activities.
6 Increasing input into a broader sphere of higher level of health care delivery system.
7 Increasing confidence in the integration of the role components.

This proposed pattern of development very much mirrored the way I saw my role developing. As the newly established clinical nurse specialist I planned to spend part of my week on both the acute and rehabilitation stroke units, and to see as many patients with strokes in the rest of the hospital as I could. My post was hospital-based, but I saw myself as a resource for community nurses who might want advice. My reflections on the relationship between the CNS and ward sister roles are outlined below.

Reflections on the CNS and ward sister roles

Pembrey (1980) sees no conflict between the role of the CNS and ward sister because the roles are organizationally different and probably complementary.

The ward sister represents continuity of nursing and social organization.

The CNS role represents 'free movement' and a resource.

My CNS role did not develop as I had originally envisaged. I had imagined it would follow Holt's (1984) pattern: a gradual increase in the sphere of influence in working with nursing colleagues and staff to change the nursing care of patients within the specialization.

Because the CNS works closely with a ward team s/he is dependent on there being a fit between the management styles of the ward sister and the specialist nurse. Furthermore, with some specialties, like the care of stroke patients, because the CNS is dealing with the whole ethos of care, and not just one aspect (such as a stoma) s/he has to be ward-based and have territorial power. Good supporting staff are also required and the CNS needs to have collaborative control with the F and E grades of patient management. Good relationships and a shared philosophy with the ward sister are crucial. Being ward-based and working with the ward team in this way has a number of advantages. The CNS has an acknowledged leadership role and credibility as a working member of a team which enables her/him to develop protocols and try out new ideas more easily as an insider rather than an outsider.

As I describe below I found myself in an unhappy situation whereby although I was ward-based, I was not accepted by the the resident ward sister and her team. This situation was not resolved for several months. Then, when the new DNS was finally appointed she insisted that the stroke patients be nursed together in a separate bay. She split the nursing establishment to provide the stroke patients with an independent nursing team. Once the separate bay was established and I had a base and a clearly delineated sphere of influence, all was much better and I was finally able to begin to develop my role following the pattern described by Holt (1984).

The need for a specialist nurse to care for people with strokes and their families is evident from the complexity of their needs as a client group.

People with strokes

People with strokes and their families are usually disadvantaged within the district general hospital with no specialist stroke services. The disabilities that have resulted from their stroke often go unrecognized. Sometimes, as long as they are continent, can walk and eat and answer uncomplicated questions put to them by nursing and medical staff, they are deemed fit for discharge, with follow-up by their GP and in the medical outpatient's department some weeks or months later.

Such a case history was brought to my attention recently by a nurse specialist colleague. Mr X was a retired gentleman, in his sixties, previously fit, living at home with his wife. His stroke necessitated admission to his local hospital where he stayed for five days. His wife, concerned and worried for him, with no other commitments at home, spent most of the hospital day with him. She helped him wash, dress and shave. 'The nurses were so busy, dear, it was the least I could do. I wanted to look after him, and I knew that I could give him more time than they could.'

So, what she called oddities of his behaviour – his memory and concentration impairment, his tendency to be so easily distracted, getting his clothes muddled when he tried to dress himself – went largely unnoticed. She did point out, she said, that he 'wasn't himself' but was told that this would get better in time.

Within a week he seemed fit enough to leave hospital and if an occupational therapist assessment had been planned to assess his spatial and perceptual difficulties, he left before it could be done.

Once home, his wife worried about his lack of progress and persistent inability to manage daily living activities without her help. She contacted her GP, who merely told her that 'it was early days yet', and hoped that the planned outpatient's appointment would provide some explanation, and pointers towards practical help.

Her husband had been driving up to the time of his stroke and she had grave doubts about how safe he would be now. But when she asked the doctor for his opinion, when the time for the outpatient's appointment finally came, he seemed to think driving no problem and breezily gave Mr X permission to go ahead. His wife confided to me several weeks later that not only would she never have dreamed of allowing her husband behind the wheel of a car, but that she realized now that there were strict regulations governing when, after a stroke, patients can recommence driving.

Although the cause of the stroke had been correctly diagnosed as atrial fibrillation and her husband was appropriately treated (with anticoagulants to minimize the risk of further embolic infarction) she was quite dissatisfied with what she perceived as a lack of knowledge about the effects a stroke could have. She felt that she was denied information and resources. A friend finally gave her the phone number of the Stroke Association, who advised her to contact the Stroke Home Rehabilitation team in her area. Ironically Mr and Mrs X lived within the catchment area of an excellent team, comprising nurse, physiotherapist, occupational therapist and speech and language therapist who subsequently gave Mrs X all the help and information she needed.

I hoped that with the establishment of the Acute Stroke Unit, the prospect of this sort of event in our hospital would become a thing of the past. I had cause, over the next few months, to reflect on why this group of patients seemed to represent such a problem. How much of the answer lay with the patients themselves and how much with the management style of the ward? Stockwell (1984) found that very few of the reasons given for nurses preferring to look after certain patients related to their nursing needs. Those they enjoyed caring for cooperated in getting well and were able to communicate readily with the nurses. They knew the nurses' names and laughed and joked with them.

Johnson and Webb (1995) consider the anthropological perspective of gift exchange, whereby patients have a limited repertoire of gifts to offer nurses, but these include the ability to contribute to ward work to make nursing work less stressful. Using the sociology of work perspective, the authors compare nurses' assessment of patients with a job interview. Not only do nurses gather biological and medical facts about their patients, they also make an assessment of their abilities to contribute to the social functioning of the ward and this plays a part in the construction of socially evaluative labels. Johnson and Webb's research, which was undertaken on one medical ward, found that the majority of nurses were aware of their judgemental approach to patients, but however guilty it made them feel, the use of evaluative labels was an important aspect of managing interpersonal relations. Despite their colleagues' friendliness and approachability even staff nurses felt they could not challenge the dominant concept of a patient's social worth. Student nurses, with their experience of different ward cultures, were also aware of the process of negative labelling and its potential to affect both the quality and intensity of care. Students were more likely to start out seeing things from the patients' rather than the staff's perspective (Smith, 1992). They were less willing than trained staff to accept labels and stereotypes but found it difficult to resist their hierarchial superiors' opinion on patients. Even when they disagreed, the ward-management style might prevent them from offering alternative perspectives.

Medical input into the care of patients with newly diagnosed stroke is relatively small by comparison with many other acute conditions. The patient's risk factors are identified and treated and their medical condition stabilized. But their rate of recovery is not always predictable and is as dependent on nursing and therapy care as it is on medical intervention.

Successful nursing management rests on a philosophy that recognizes the following factors:

- That a proportion of stroke patients are bound to fall into the 'unpopular' classification. That is, they are unable to communicate or laugh and joke with the nurses and they do not 'cooperate' in getting well (Stockwell, 1984). Those with a left-sided hemiplegia and cognitive impairment are likely to deny their problems and have little insight into how disabled they are.
- That care has to be assessed and planned from the patient's perspective, rather than that of the nurses and doctors.
- That an enquiring and analytical approach to nursing care is essential. Staff have to be able to recognize the patients' and carers' problems; to recognize what problems these will pose for the nurses; and to identify and utilize all the resources available in order to make nursing management less daunting.

When we had patients on the Acute Stroke Unit who were unconscious, they usually had anxious relatives and friends who needed explanations and sympathy. When patients' memory and cognitive abilities were impaired I asked their relatives to bring in photographs and reminders of what sort of characters they were. One of the most difficult things in relationships with both the patients and relatives was the fact that the staff had no conception of how the newly disabled person had been, before the stroke. It took time to build up a picture of just who this person was. Patients who came back to visit us when I was running the medical ward and rehabilitation unit would comment on the importance of this aspect of their care. James, in his early forties, with a young family, whose stroke had left him with a dense left-sided weakness, described it as 'crucial'. After his stroke he felt devastated, his self-esteem and sense of self as low as it could be. The fact that the staff worked hard to recognize his previous strengths and abilities, and saw him as a whole person, despite his limitations was, he claimed, a major factor in his recovery.

Acknowledging patients' and relatives' distress and answering their questions was a very necessary part of care on the new unit. The project that the purchasers had initiated had revealed that lack of information about what was happening was seen by newly diagnosed stroke patients and their relatives as one of their greatest frustrations. In the first few weeks they rarely required detailed explanations of what a stroke was or why it had happened; simply, knowledge of the care being given, the immediate plans and the short-term goals.

As discussed in the next section, good nursing documentation is an important vehicle for addressing some of the complexities associated with caring for people with strokes and their families.

Documentation

Nursing has a strong oral narrative tradition. A wealth of events and decisions which happen to and around patients are communicated between staff within the course of a shift. However, when it comes to passing on information in a written form nurses have a tendency to interpret, rather than directly record the facts (Street, 1992). I remember early on in my career as a ward sister nursing an angry elderly lady who would not take her medication, despite all our persuasive efforts. The medical staff needed to be convinced that we were dealing with someone who adamantly refused the treatment they had prescribed. Her behaviour had been briefly summarized in nursing reports as being aggressive and uncooperative; but one evening after she had thrown her toilet bag across the ward, upturned a full bowl of water on to a staff nurse and directed a few choice words of verbal abuse at her, we decided to record these events exactly.

By the time the next ward round took place, several such incidents had been described which we read out to the doctors. Only then were they able to realize our difficulties in looking after her and, in the light of this, decided to review the treatment they had prescribed. This factual, descriptive evidence enabled doctors and nurses to reflect together on what the problems were and how to overcome them.

Street (1992) observes how nursing notes rarely reflect the patients' view of the world or an articulated picture of the clinical care; and so the nursing care provided remains invisible. Nurses document basic information about the work completed but fail in accurately communicating the nature of their work (Howse and Bailey, 1992). The subordinate role of nursing care may be linked to difficulties in expressing the nature of nursing practice (Ekman and Segesten, 1995).

Hart (1991) comments on how highly articulate nurses are in the way they express their views informally among their peers. Yet there is a reluctance among nurses to express their views more formally or commit them to paper. This can be ascribed to difficulties in finding exact definitions and lack of confidence in writing (Howse and Bailey, 1992; Ekman and Segesten, 1995). Inflexibility of documentation and the time it takes inhibit writing. So do social factors, such as established group-work norms, and work values which protect the group members from the demand to carry out tasks they consider to be unrewarding (Howse and Bailey, 1995). Added to this, nurses have a tendency not to read their colleagues' nursing notes.

In the newly established stroke unit, it was agreed between the ward sister and myself that care plans which the students or junior staff nurses and I wrote together when we were looking after the stroke patients should be left at the end of each bed. I explained the importance of instant accessibility to handling and swallowing instructions for this vulnerable group of patients. Invariably when I returned to the ward they had been carefully put away in plastic covers inside a file that was kept at the nursing station. Only when I attended handovers and took them with me, were they used for reflecting on and evaluating care.

This compared strikingly with the way in which I had been accustomed to using documentation. Within my own ward it had been seen as a necessary adjunct to verbal communication and the only way of avoiding communication breakdowns within a shift system where key people could be off-duty when vital information was needed. We also regarded it as a time-saving device. Although we had daily verbal updates with the other members of the multidisciplinary team, at other times, when an interruption would be awkward for either nurses or patients, we would direct the staff towards the folder at the end of the patient's bed and request that they read, rather than be told, about the patient's progress. Similarly, we taught some of the team members to write down progress reviews and new instructions when there was no nurse available to speak to, and just to remind us to read them. Eventually, it became an accepted part of ward practice for the documentation to contain information from the therapists and social workers as well as from ward nurses and specialist nurses. However, it took time to evaluate the effectiveness of the care given, and to review the plans.

Staff learned to snatch odd moments for writing and for updating charts: while they were sitting supervising patients' meals, or overseeing them practise daily living activities. However, the time taken allowed us flexibility. Members of staff who were owed hours could take them back on quieter days as soon as they had finished their morning's work. Their updated documentation meant that another member of the team, even a relatively junior student, could speak for them at handovers. Time-consuming instructions to trained agency staff who arrived after the shift had started were avoided when we judged them able to manage by just being introduced to their allocated patients and reading their care plans.

Documentation wasn't always done perfectly; and like every nurse, we were all guilty of not always reading what others wrote. Nonetheless, by believing in its importance as a working tool, a philosophy developed that saw accurate charting and written problem identification, planning and evaluating as vital to the way we nursed.

This philosophy made a difference to our sense of ourselves as nurses. It made invisible work visible by showing the 'working out'. By detailing the steps involved in attaining goals we were able to reflect back, to recognize what our achievements had been and make them evident to other team members. As well as recording patients' needs and when they were resolved, we were critical and questioning on paper. It was common to find 'why?' written in a care plan, which stimulated discussion of how nurses had arrived at decisions they made about the patient's care.

I found nursing documentation an invaluable teaching tool. The high workload on the ward and the under-establishment of permanent staff allowed very little time for formal teaching sessions. Writing care plans with students and newly qualified nurses gave space for reflection, for questioning and musing about nursing and the patients.

It also enabled me to emphasize how important it was to give credence to the patient's feelings as well as to the problems and challenges they presented. We would include in the care an awareness, for instance, of the embarrassment a patient might feel about their incontinence, or their anger and frustration about having lost their ability to get out of bed unaided and how this might affect their recovery and their attitudes towards the staff.

Access to the documentation by patients and relatives made us particularly aware of our accountability. We had to be able to justify what we wrote and this eliminated any inclination to be judgemental or stray from the facts. The nursing notes, apart from the page that gave personal information and the medical diagnosis, were kept at the end of the beds, and on occasions were read by the patients and their relatives. We made it clear that we encouraged them to write, too, and the communication sheet contained our reminders about bringing in their father's slippers, or theirs that 'Mum would like to see the chiropodist'; but sometimes we came across gratifying comments about how the relatives appreciated all we were doing and the nursing team would feel quite uplifted.

End thoughts

1   Resolution of communication breakdowns depends on improving documentation systems (Howse and Bailey, 1992). Practical measures to improve accessibility are important, as is an understanding of the factors and processes that affect documentation such as how it is valued

as a work activity. If problems persist, they are to the detriment of patients and nursing.

2   Nurse educators have a part to play in improving documentation. A big theory–practice gap potentially exists if lecturers are not sufficently familiar with how ward nurses document the evaluation of their care. Without this familiarization, teaching is likely to result in students writing 'essays' on ward documentation which do not incorporate the essence of the nursing care given. Wards with good documentation systems therefore could be identified by educators to assist them to initiate practice-led teaching.

3   Documentation has to make sense to all nurses and to be seen as a valuable activity. One possible way forward is to involve the multi-disciplinary team in collaborative care-planning as described elsewhere in this chapter. Another way forward is the use of critical pathways as a documentation framework. Critical pathways have the potential for 'variance analysis' which gives nurses the opportunity to track the content of their care and reflect on the factors which intervened to prevent it from not going according to plan (Wigfield and Boon, 1996). The value of this approach is that nurses are able to document the factors which intervened to prevent them from achieving a planned task. Nurses often have the intention of carrying out a certain activity but the unpredictable nature of ward work may mean that other priorities take over. Documenting these situations may mean that nurses are able to define and identify more exactly the nature of the care they give.

4   In line with current health service trends, documentation can be seen as a form of evidence-based nursing by which processes and outcomes are 'detailed' and solutions to problems produced.

Documentation is an important component of the communication system for ensuring and auditing quality patient care. However, the written word needs to be informed by verbal handovers which together provide a mechanism for problem-solving and reflection, which is the theme of the next section.

Handovers, problem-solving and reflection

For most patients, hospitalization within a medical (rather than a surgical) ward is an unsought, unwelcome and transient part of their life. My aim was always to keep their stay to a minimum, by anticipating their nursing needs. Having worked with elderly patients for much of my career I was also aware of the fact that as they get better, they can 'peak': that is, reach a level at which they are fit for discharge, but then deteriorate and become prey to iatrogenic infections if leaving hospital is delayed for non-medical reasons.

To facilitate a timely discharge, we needed as rounded a view of the patient as possible and we needed to develop clear goals. Shift handovers were the time when nurses had an opportunity to pool their ideas about patients and their care, and reflect on and evaluate nursing actions. Handovers are an important and much-researched part of nursing. They can be used thoughtfully as a basis for reflective practice, where both patients' problems and nurses' problems with patients are mulled over and refined (McMahon, 1991; Smith, 1992). Within my ward area, handovers were used as a forum for communication and for updating events within an ever-changing environment. They were an opportunity to gather data about how different people nursed and interpreted their role. Critical incidents were examined and comparisons made with past management.

Questions were asked such as: 'Why did he have such a bad night? Is he in pain, worried, confused? What could be causing the confusion? Is there an indication for night sedation?' Solutions were brainstormed and nursing care was prescribed. We identified resources that could help us solve the problems. These could be people, with appropriate knowledge or skills, or equipment. Working with stroke patients could involve detailed discussion about moving and handling techniques and we shared information and used past experiences to work out what would be most effective. Another resource was the library, and a photocopy of relevant research would be put in the patient's folder alongside their nursing documentation to back up the rationale for decisions or to stimulate discussion.

Another important function of the nursing handover was role-modelling and teaching nurses to be proactive. I felt that it was important for them to realize just how active a part they could play in the patient's recovery and not see themselves merely as instruments of other disciplines, passively taking a caretaking role while others healed the patient (McMahon, 1991). For this reason, a necessary part of handing over care to the nurses on the next shift was being aware of the overall plan, and when discharge from hospital was likely. An aspect that to me seemed vital was the inclusion of the opinions of all grades of staff. We all had different perspectives on the patients which depended on either who we were, or when we saw them. All the nursing staff were a resource whose different experiences of the same people helped to complete the picture of them and their needs. The more information there was, the easier it was to identify the problems and to find solutions.

However, handover sessions can be fraught with difficulties. Not all ward areas contain space where nurses can't be overheard discussing patients; yet moving beyond sight of the patients limits the number of nurses who can participate. There is always a time constraint, interruptions can be numerous and the balance constantly has to be weighed between discussing patients' needs and nurses' feelings. The overlap between shifts is often the only opportunity within the working day or night for nurses to unburden themselves of the stress their work has caused them. At times only a small fraction of the issues raised can be dealt with; some are picked up later on, some inevitably get lost. At their best, shift handovers are a stimulating way of promoting nursing as positive, questioning and non-judgemental. They are an ideal opportunity for giving positive feedback and for being seen to condone its use. They are an opportunity to raise nurses' self-esteem and to unify and motivate a team. At their worst, they do little more than provide a retrospective account of the patient's medical condition, and condone labelling and stereotyping as a way of dealing with the problems that are presented.

A problem-solving patient-centred approach to care has been seen as one of the most important changes in nursing over the last decade. Nurses, however, need to have acquired skills in reflective practice and problem identification in order to be able to pick out problems that may not be obvious, and in which they can be emotionally involved (Dewing, 1990). Hurst, Dean and Trickey (1991), in researching nurses' problem-solving behaviour, found it a poorly understood feature of modern nursing. Nurses use a variety of problem-solving processes. They might just recall a solution from memory or they might use trial and error until a successful outcome is achieved. However, when following a stages model of problem-solving, the researchers found that nurses concentrated on the 'doing' aspects at the expense of the analytical process associated with planning and evaluation. Their literature review revealed that evaluation is the least understood and least used stage in clinical problem-solving. In their own study they found that the majority of nurses didn't see evaluation as important. Because of the complex nature of stroke patients' disabilities, I considered reflection and problem-solving to be an essential feature of their care and discharge planning.

I needed all my personal and nursing skills which I have just described to see me through what was to be a traumatic transition of setting up a new Stroke Unit.

The ideals and challenges of the new Stroke Unit

Following the closure and disestablishment of my own ward and the relocation of a new Stroke Unit in another ward (i.e. a Unit within an already-existing medical ward), we needed to build up another team of nurses who could, with guidance and education from me, develop their skills in looking after stroke patients. Sadly, it was to be a long time before this eventually happened. The setting up of the new Unit was intensely traumatic for all concerned. Those who were keen to promote more skilled and knowledgeable care of the stroke patients had to deal with the anger, antagonism and rejection of these patients by the sister into whose ward the Unit had to be incorporated. Why was the ward sister so unwilling to take on this group of patients? The 'top down' imposition of the change and the fact that it was created by the hospital management were important factors. Another was the absence by this time, and for the next few months, of a permanent nurse manager to support and guide her through a difficult time: the ward had already been relocated some months before when the medical unit was reorganized.

There were still vacancies on the rota and this caused a lot of anxiety about how heavy the workload would be. The inevitability of the change and repeated explanations that the purchasers had been insistent on its establishment well before the Unit was actually set up, didn't affect her views. Nor did pointing out how this was the only possible geographical location for the Stroke Unit, since the other medical wards contained specialist units with purpose-built housing or equipment. She still maintained that 'The stroke patients should be on another ward.' It had been made clear that unlike the patients on the rehabilitation unit, now housed in another part of the hospital, those on the acute Stroke Unit would not all be heavy. A proportion of the eight allocated beds would be taken by patients with mild strokes who would be there to benefit from the concentrated therapy input and the time and education that could be given to them by the specialist nurse. These were patients, therefore, who would not require an excessive amount of the ward staff's time.

The extra resources that had been allocated were emphasized: a clinical nurse specialist, increased input from the therapists, and a social worker to work mostly with the stroke patients. The nursing staff were not unused to looking after this speciality; all the wards on the medical wing took stroke patients within 24 hours of their admission; and the ward's nursing establishment now included trained staff very experienced in managing people with strokes, who were more than ready to use and share their skills.

The management style of the ward where the acute Stroke Unit was placed was one that used a biomedical approach to care, rather than a nursing process, patient-centred philosophy. The importance of the ward nursing style had not been recognized by the management team when planning the Unit; it was glibly assumed that the presence of the clinical nurse specialist and the incorporation into the team of nurses skilled in caring for stroke patients, would be sufficient to ensure that nursing care met the patients' needs.

As stated towards the end of the previous section, because of the complex nature of the stroke patients' disabilities I considered reflection and problem-solving to be an essential feature of their care and discharge-planning. On the ward in which the acute Stroke Unit had been placed there was no culture of reflection, evaluation nor of looking forward towards discharge. Indeed, on one occasion when I suggested that the social worker and occupational therapist be informed of a patient's improvement so that we could modify our plans, one of the more senior members of nursing staff looked at me in amazement with the comment: 'but the doctors haven't said anything yet about this patient going home.'

Nurses on the Unit who spent most time doing emotional work with these patients and their relatives were those who had previously worked with the rehabilitating stroke patients and saw it as an integral part of their role. One of these nurses, a well-organized worker, and a skilled and empathetic communicator, was criticized by the ward sister for 'spending too much time chatting and not pulling her weight'. Though emotional care was done on the ward and noticed by other staff, it was seen as secondary rather than complementary to the physical work and was not examined or discussed by the ward sister. Even though it was recognized to be a part of the CNS role it was not seen as working and was viewed negatively: 'All the patients will think they are going to be treated like that.' Smith (1992) maintains that the importance of defining care as work cannot be under-estimated: that this most essential ingredient of what nurses do apart from being recognized and valued, should be supported educationally and organizationally.

Lack of constructive discussion about the nurses' and patients' feelings made for an atmosphere where positive feedback and praise for achieve-ments was difficult to give and often rejected. On one occasion when I tried to convey a family's thanks for the care the nurses had given their relative, I was cut short by the ward sister, voicing a presumption that they wanted to make a complaint.

My intention of sharing my years of clinical skills, my knowledge and experience in nursing stroke patients, with another area, was dependent on there being some fit between the culture and atmosphere I had created in my own ward, described in the first section of this chapter, and the area in which I was currently working.

The definition of nursing, within the two areas, however, was radically different. Just as I found features of the ward unsympathetic and not conducive to my style of caring, so, to the ward sister and her team, I represented a change in nursing style that they were not prepared to countenance. These differences were not rooted in formal education. A large proportion of the team working on the Acute Stroke Unit were nurses qualified within the last ten years who had been brought up on a nursing process philosophy and the concept of individualized patient care. Nearly all of them were either studying for a post-registration qualification, or had recently completed a course of study. The ward sister had a relevant degree and was currently doing a management diploma. There was a determina-tion to preserve their way of working despite role-modelling from forces on the inside and outside and the advent of a group of patients whose management they could have made easier.

Why did the ward sister prove so effective in stalling the development of the new Unit? Part of the answer lies in the nature of her power and the characteristics of the nursing workforce.

The power of the ward sister and the characteristics of the nursing workforce

The ward sister has power that is strong enough to resist attempts to modify her management style or make changes on her ward: even in the face of pressure from her peer groups, medical staff and general management as representatives of the purchasers. Lewis (1990), in exploring ward sisters' perceptions of their responsibilities, describes them as the group who effectively control how the profession of nursing is carried out. Activities sanctioned by ward sisters are legitimized as appropriate nursing behaviour. By virtue of their appointment and their position they are able to negate any efforts to bring changes into nursing.

There are various sources of the ward sister's power: she chooses her staff nurses who become her culture-bearers. If the staff have worked within the hospital, or been students on the sister's ward, they are likely to be sympathetic to her philosophy and style. If they are unfamiliar with the ward, they are liable to conform to group norms (Stockwell, 1984) or to leave. The ward sister who resists change, who is inclined to act passively and think negatively, attracts a like-minded group of staff to an environment which remains static. Those who welcome stimulation and change, who see facilitating growth and development as an important part of their role, choose staff who ask questions and seek a rationale for their actions; who are not afraid to challenge and can provide research-based answers when questioned.

At the present time, with so many unfilled nursing vacancies within the National Health Service (particularly in large cities) there is little pressure on staff to stay in a job they do not enjoy. Even if there are aspects of a ward's style that nurses feel unhappy with, their ability of adaptability enables them to work around it. Nurses' adaptability is both their strength and their weakness: a strength because they manage the demands of shift work, working different hours each day, different days each week and coping with last minute alterations to the rota. They deal with an ever-changing group of patients and with regular rotations of virtually all the staff who work with them. Their priorities are constantly being rethought during the course of a working day, as unforeseen emergencies and unexpected events occur. They are constantly making order out of the chaos that is an inevitable part of the acute hospital ward.

Nurses' adaptability is also their weakness because they can unquestioningly adopt dubious or outdated work practices. Some years ago when I was facilitating the introduction of the nursing process philosophy into a ward which was managed on a task-allocation basis, I came across a student I had worked with. She was just qualifying and her only previous experience of task allocation had been as part of nursing history; yet she complied unprotestingly with this outmoded way of managing patient care.

'You get used to it,' she told me. Nurses' adaptability works against them as far as general management is concerned: because they are able to fill in for other roles – for domestic and medical shortages – their multiple, inter-changeable skills are seen as evidence that they are unspecialized. This translates in workload studies as nurses having skills that are easily transferable. Their expertise in caring remains invisible (Hart, 1991).

The ward sister decides what nursing is on her ward. She defines the principles that rule nursing actions. She sets the standards and monitors competence (Lewis, 1990) and so determines the nature of nursing; she decides how staff should spend their time and fits the task to the person; she sets the emotional tone of the ward (Smith, 1992). The conditions she creates determine what depth of care is given to the patients and staff. In developing her staff she can instill into them her vision and awareness of what nursing can achieve. Staff who have regular performance reviews and objectives set and discussed, whose achievements are praised and recognized, develop a sense of nursing as a valued and accountable profession. They learn to recognize their potential for autonomy and control.

The ward sister who has budgetary control decides on the skill mix (Roberts, 1993). One of the ways in which she can support her staff on a day-to-day basis, even when she doesn't see them, is by ensuring that the rota contains an appropriate mix of experienced and inexperienced staff. This enables them to learn from one another and their confidence grows. Without the right skill mix, staff can feel they have been deserted.

The ward sister acts as the gatekeeper (Lewis, 1990) and manages the interface between all the agencies, groups and professionals who deal with the patient (Pembrey, 1980; Hart, 1991). She controls communication coming in and out of the ward, as well as within the ward; as the manager of the interface she acts as a reference point, a representative and an inter-preter. In creating the atmosphere of the ward she influences how welcome or receptive it is to other members of the multidisciplinary team. She can encourage or discourage collaborative working practices.

Thoughts for the future: adapting to the changing health service

The ward sister is still the key to nursing. If ward sisters are role models of a style of nursing that adversely effects patient care, managers have to know about it and to be strong, skilled and interested enough to put it right.

Nurse managers are very important in overseeing the quality of sisters and avoiding the situation I faced when I had to work with a colleague whose practice had gone unchecked over many years. This situation should now be more easily monitored as there is more audit going on: for example, wards have to submit performance indicators, including documentation audit, skill mix and the use of agency staff. Even though this is quantitative data, its presentation requires the ward sister to share information. This makes the ward's clinical practice public, when previously it had been her sole and impenetrable domain.

Managing the budget has become one of the essential components of a ward sister's job. There is scope for creative working patterns in order that the most expensive resource – the staff – is used wisely, for example, 'twilight shifts' or shifts that accommodate working parents, rather than everyone coming and going at the same time. These changes would depend on excellent communication systems incorporating good documentation.

These new accounting practices mean that nurses need to be aware of the part research skills play in the day-to-day mangement of the ward. They have to learn how to evaluate their own practice from the inside and see how it can facilitate patient care. External audit alone is not the answer, but approaches such as 'variance analysis' previously described, as part of evidence-based nursing, offers one way forward.

It is important that there is a strong nursing voice within general management which represents and incorporates the views of frontline nurses. Directors of Nursing Services (DNS) have to have enough power to do this and to make a difference. For example, the combination of the DNS who is also an assistant general manager can be particularly powerful in promoting better understanding of the links between management and nursing.

Coda on contracting: you don't know what you've got until it's gone

Savage (1995) whose research project explored the therapeutic potential of nurses' personal involvement with patients and the notion of 'closeness' describes how 'in writing up the study I set out to record something that has been lost'. 'Sweeping changes' had occurred and Jones Ward, which had previously practised a form of nursing which conformed to Manthey's (1992) definition of primary nursing had 'changed beyond recognition'. The frequent changes in location, inadequate staffing levels, increased non-nursing duties and/or quasi-medical tasks resulted in stress and dissatisfaction. Many staff left, including all the primary nurses, and the flattened hierarchy gave way to a 'more traditional hierarchy with a ward sister in overall charge'. I could identify with Savage's description in relation to my own situation and the majority of hospitals over the last decade.

Three issues emerged for me from Savage's description. These were the potentially demoralizing effect of changes in location; the increase in quasi-medical tasks undertaken by nurses; and a culture change.

With regard to changes in location, ward moves are increasingly becoming a part of hospital life as a result of cost-reduction programmes. A strong nursing voice is required to ensure that nurses work in suitable environ-ments and that they have sufficent space and adequate facilities to ensure safe ward storage and good housekeeping. As areas are shut, nurses need to find ways of preventing patients from being relocated into buildings which do not have facilities to nurse them. A suitable environment is one of the tools of the nurse's trade. Without being able to control it they will be subject to unnecessary stress and frustrations which waste valuable energy.

Taking on quasi-medical tasks may have implications in terms of the skill mix of ward establishments. Nurses therefore have to be able to provide evidence as to why a more senior member of staff may be required. For example, the introduction of night nursing practitioners rather than unit-based night sisters may mean that nurses don't get the support at night that they used to have. The comforting night sister role is less in evidence since she spends more of her time taking on some of the tasks previously undertaken by junior doctors, such as recannulating, doing ECG's and certifying expected deaths.

This situation requires enough seniority in the nurse running the ward to be able to manage without being dependent on much input from the night practitioner which has superseded the night sister's role.

The change in culture has a number of dimensions. Wards are much busier now, with bed occupancy sometimes as much as 97 per cent. In some hospitals Interim Care Units offer hostel-like facilities to accommodate patients who were previously 'up and about' and practically ready to go home. These are the patients who were an important source of support which is now denied to the ward sister, nurses and other patients.

Take Frank, a teacher in his late forties who had developed good relationships with the staff and other patients and offered understanding and support. A quick comment as we went to take his blood pressure, showed that he could see and appreciate the emotional labour being undertaken by staff and how hard it was to maintain. By recognizing how we cared for the patients, Frank articulated for us the value of giving emotional support. An interchange went on between us and Frank which allowed recognition of how difficult it was to care. The complaint in the letter referred to at the beginning of this chapter shows how staff, who did not value or recognize emotional labour, blocked any dialogue with anxious relatives about their mothers.

> discussions with the nursing staff, either when we visited the ward, or by telephone always resulted in defensive comments about the care she was receiving, and there was very little concern for her general well-being or how her relatives were feeling. When we expressed our worries, or made sugges-tions, the response from the nurses was very negative.

This response demonstrates what Kirkpatrick (1967) recognized 30 years ago: that there is a real need to teach support and to encourage communication. 'Without it the nurse feels unwanted and anyone who feels unwanted becomes apathetic towards all those in [his] care ... Nurses need to be cared for and to be recognised as individuals' (p. 52).

The ward sister's emotional labour is closely related to that of her staff. If she recognizes the nurses as individuals, they in turn feel cared for and wanted. They are then enabled to create the 'caring and loving environment' which allows patients (like the subject of the letter) to make 'a remarkable recovery'.

References

Aradine C R and Denyes, M J (1972) Activities and pressures of clinical nurse specialists. *Nursing Research* 21 (5): 411–19.

Boucher A and Bruce S (1972) *Similarities and Differences in the Role of the Clinical Nurse Specialist*. American Nurse Association, 8th Research Conference: 163–87.

Castledine G (1982) The role and function of clinical nurse specialists in England and Wales. MSc thesis, University of Manchester.

Castledine G (1995) Defining specialist nursing (editorial). *British Journal of Nursing* 4 (5).

Department of Health (1992) *Health of the Nation: A Strategy for Health in England*. HMSO, London.

Dewing J (1990) Reflective Practice. *Senior Nurse* 10: 26–8.

Ekman I and Segesten K (1995) Deputed power of medical control: The hidden message in the ritual of oral shift reports. *Journal of Advanced Nursing* 22: 1006–11.

Fineman S (1993) Organisations as emotional arenas. In Fineman S (ed.) *Emotion in Organisations*. Sage, London.

Fretwell J E (1982) *Ward Teaching and Learning: Sister and the Learning Environment*. RCN, London.

Hart E (1991) Ghost in the machine. *Health Services Journal* 101: 20–2.

Holt F M (1984) A theoretical model for specialist practice. *Nursing and Health Care* 5: 447–9.

Howse E and Bailey J (1992) Resistance to documentation – a nursing research issue. *International Journal of Nursing Studies* 29 (4): 371–80.

Hurst K, Dean A and Trickey S (1991) The recognition and non-recognition of problem-solving stages in nursing practice. *Journal of Advanced Nursing* 16: 1444–55.

Johnson M and Webb C (1995) Rediscovering unpopular patients: The concept of social judgment. *Journal of Advanced Nursing* 21: 466–75.

Kirkpatrick W J A (1967) Conscience and commitment. In Robb B *Sans Everything. A Case to Answer*. Nelson, London.

Lewis T (1990) The hospital ward sister: professional gatekeeper. *Journal of Advanced Nursing* 15: 808–18.

Manthey M (1992) *The Practice of Primary Nursing*. King's Fund Centre, London.

McMahon R (1991) Therapeutic nursing: theories, issues and practice. In McMahon R and Pearson A (eds) *Nursing as Therapy*. Chapman & Hall, London.

Ogier M (1982) *An Ideal Sister*. RCN, London.

Pembrey S E M (1980) *The Ward Sister – Key to Nursing*. RCN, London.

Roberts J (1993) The G grade ward sister: clinical expert and ward manager. *British Journal of Nursing* 2 (4): 242–7.

Savage J (1995) *Nursing Intimacy*. Scutari Press, London.

Smith M (1990) Making the most of the CNS. *Senior Nurse* 10 (9): 6–8.

Smith P (1992) *The Emotional Labour of Nursing*. Macmillan, London.

Stockwell F (1972, reprinted 1984) *The Unpopular Patient*. Croom Helm, Beckenham.

Strauss A, Fagerhaugh S, Suczek B and Wiener C (1982) Sentimental work in the technologised hospital. *Sociology of Health and Illness* 4 (3): 254–78.

Street A F (1992) *Inside Nursing: A Critical Ethnography in Clinical Nursing Practice*. State University of New York, Albany.

United Kingdom Central Council for Nursing, Midwifery and Health Visiting (1994) *The Future of Professional Practice – the Council's Standards for Education and Practice following Registration*. UKCC, London.

Wigfield and Boon (1996) Critical care pathway development: the way forward. *British Journal of Nursing* 5: 12.

Wilson–Barnett J (1986) Ethical dilemmas in nursing. *Journal of Medical Ethics* 12: 123–6, 135.

Wilson–Barnett J (1995) Specialism in nursing: effectiveness and maximisation of benefit. *Journal of Advanced Nursing* 21: 1–2.

9

Nursing Development Units: perspectives and prospects for research and practice

Anne Jones and Olwyn Bamford

Nothing is more difficult than to know precisely what we see. (Merleau-Ponty, 1962, p. 58)

In this chapter the two authors describe and analyse their collective experience of creating an environment in which change, and the setting up of a Nursing Development Unit was possible. They worked closely together for six years and the experiences documented in the chapter span that time. It begins with an overview of the background to the development of Nursing Development Units (NDUs) in general and their NDU in particular. They then focus on the steps taken within their own area in bringing about and sustaining changes which allowed them to designate their ward as an NDU. They also identify some of the hidden issues which allowed them to proceed and succeed. A major part of the chapter then explores their experience of generating knowledge through practice and research undertaken by themselves and others. They consider the relationship of practice, research and development in their own setting and how to make it meaningful to other practitioners.

Introduction

We chose the introductory quotation to illustrate some of the difficulties we faced while writing the chapter. The embodiment of our knowledge and experiences meant that often we felt unable to recognize the developments and achievements we wished to describe. In a sense we had to undertake an anthropological process of making the familiar strange in order to reflect in an objective way. Despite much discussion and reflection, the translation of our thoughts into typescript seemed at times an impossibility. Our concerns included the dilemma of whether to recreate our memories at all, or whether to leave our stories untold. We often convinced ourselves the latter option was more sensible as our recollections were accompanied by various emotions, many of them painful. Indeed, for that reason, an original group of five contributors dwindled over the months, leaving only the two of us. However, we have long felt the need to share our story with a wider audience, perhaps to make some contribution to the collective knowledge and understanding of nursing. We have tried to present an honest and candid account and hope we have done justice to the creativity, innovation, commitment and motivation that we shared with so many patients and colleagues along the way.

As frontline practitioners we held a fundamental belief that the most experienced ward nurses should be those providing direct patient care, acting as role models to facilitate student learning and the development of more junior qualified staff, and be easily available as information resources. Through our work on a Nursing Development Unit we were constantly exploring the relationship between our environment and the knowledge and practice of nursing. In retrospect we see that our NDU and others like it had created a new agenda for nursing. These units legitimized the knowledge and practice of nursing and facilitated innovations like primary nursing. In the context of this book, therefore, Nursing Development Units can be seen as being implicated in the setting of new agendas for nursing research, and in particular for practice-based research. However, in order for these new agendas to be taken forward and promoted, support is required, in the same way that continued support is required to develop and sustain NDUs in the first place. Large-scale managerial reorganization within the health service has caused a shift in the locus of power. Changes in power structures within hospitals has meant that support for nurses and nursing practice has changed radically, and has been perceived in some cases as having disappeared altogether.

In summary, our chapter aims to:

- Provide background on the NDU movement
- Make explicit our view that units involved in developments and challenging practice can make a major contribution to nursing
- Help other units involved in developments feel more confident and supported to promote, sell and replicate their achievements
- Put value on 'the small things' related to aspects of care, which may not have been mentioned elsewhere in the NDU literature
- Recognize 'the small things' as significant steps towards progress which provide the foundations on which to build and move forward
- Formalize our experience through writing, and create a tool to support others in their endeavours to change their nursing organization and practice.

Background

In preparing this chapter we consulted a number of people whom we had worked with in setting up and running our Nursing Development Unit. We also drew on a file full of materials from the period which included articles and funding proposals we had written.

Our first proposal was a bid to become one of the first 'official' NDUs in the country. The proposal, submitted in 1989, was a response to a scheme being set up by Jane Salvage, Director of Nursing Developments at the King's Fund, to support nursing innovation. Financial backing was provided by the Sainsbury Charitable Trust. Jane's rationale for the scheme was to help tackle government under-investment in nursing research and development which in her view had the effect that: 'nurses often lack the skill, education or opportunity to acquire expertise, to scrutinise their work or to introduce changes which may benefit patients' (Salvage, 1989). The setting up of NDUs therefore was seen as one way of rectifying this situation.

The NDU movement

The NDU movement began during the 1980s, inspired by units set up by Alan Pearson in Oxford and Steve Wright in Thameside. These units became famous for their innovative nursing practices such as primary nursing and nurse prescribing. Salvage (1989) characterized the goals of these and other NDUs as sharing:

> a commitment to practising the best possible standards of nursing, and to sharing with others the insights gained through close scrutiny of their own work. This means creating a climate which is open and questioning, and where change is almost a way of life – not for change's own sake, but as part of the ceaseless search for improvement.(p. 25)

In our own case, the sequence for change laid down in our ward action plan was based on the model used by Pearson for the introduction of primary nursing in the Burford Nursing Development Unit. A questioning approach to care was beginning to stir in the minds of staff and therefore a need to measure the quality of care both before and after the introduction of primary nursing was considered appropriate to provide more tangible evidence of its effect. This evidence, in the form of a baseline assessment with which to make future comparisons, would then be available to staff, not just on the ward but also in the rest of the hospital. The help of a local research nurse was sought to assist us undertake a quality assessment both before and one year after the change.

Once nurses had become patient-focused through the introduction of primary nursing, developments were then approached in a more systematic way. With the achievement of our initial goal – that of introducing primary nursing – staff began to see an endless list of advances they could make to improve the care they provided for patients. This period was marked with frustration: knowing what was wanted, but often not having either the time or knowledge to implement it.

The link with the research nurse led us to the belief that we had developed the ward sufficiently to make a bid to the King's Fund for funding to become an NDU.

Extracts from our King's Fund proposal

The following extracts taken from our King's Fund proposal very much capture the spirit and goals of the NDU movement expressed by Jane Salvage. The extracts also trace the development of our unit and give some indication of who we regarded as the major national and international influences on our work. With hindsight, our belief that nursing had undergone 'a great shift' from subservience to power was perhaps over optimistic. However, our belief in nursing's creativity remains steadfast. In the interests of confidentiality, we do not refer to our ward or hospital by name.

This proposal describes our progress towards a Nursing Development Unit based on an acute medical ward and our plans for the future at that time. Our mission for the NDU is summarized as:

1   to provide excellence in nursing
2   to be a focus of development for clinical practice
3   to raise the profile of nursing as a profession.

History of nursing developments on our ward

The 1980s saw a great shift in the emphasis of nursing from one of subservience to becoming a very powerful and creative discipline. Development of the clinical nursing role and a clinical career structure is now a subject of much discussion among nurses throughout the world.

The excitement generated by these many changes left us longing to be involved, but lacking the confidence and knowledge of where to begin. The work of Alan Pearson at Burford Community Hospital, and later Beeson ward at the Radcliffe Infirmary, seemed to clarify a route for us to start working towards change. In June 1986 we laid down a two-year plan to introduce primary nursing as part of our strategy for change.

We define primary nursing as care given by a designated registered nurse (RGN) who has autonomy and 24-hour accountability for a group of patients from admission to discharge. In their absence the care is carried out by an associate nurse as documented in the care plan. The elements of this definition came from Manthey (1980) and Pearson (1983).

Following a seminar on clinical developments in July 1987 by Dr Susan Pembrey at our hospital, it became apparent that many other areas were interested in change. Despite the threats of ward closures, the inspiration and enthusiasm injected by Dr Pembrey remained throughout the hospital.

Development of nursing

Our questioning approach to care has resulted in most interactions being research-based, but many of our questions remain unanswered. We are keen, therefore, to fill some of these gaps and launch our own research projects. We feel the need to develop an understanding of research theory and methods first. Obviously we are all aware that to achieve our future aims we rely on help from others. We are fortunate to be able to draw on the expertise and support of a number of local nurse researchers and teachers with whom we have worked closely in planning and implementing our research activities as outlined below.

Future research includes exploring the concept of partnership between nurse and client and the effect of not wearing a uniform. This is one indicator of the change in relationship between nurse and client. We are also planning a feasibility study on self-medication.

We plan to share our knowledge with a wider audience by providing seminars and workshops and we aim to extend the ward library as a resource for nursing developments. We are also exploring therapeutic touch, using massage, aromatherapy and reflexology (Maxwell-Hudson, 1987). We are fortunate to have several members of staff competent in some of these techniques.

Evaluation

Primary nursing is a relatively new way of organizing nursing care in Britain and to date there is not a great deal of information available on evaluation. A number of evaluation tools exist including QualPacs (Wandelt and Ager 1974). [We had carried out a number of QualPacs assessments to provide baseline data on quality of care, before the implementation of primary nursing.] Subsequent assessments showed an improvement in quality as measured by the tool. We were also able to observe a general improvement in morale among staff and patients since the implementation of primary nursing. This observation was further confirmed by low staff turnover and a reduction in the employment cost of agency nurses.

Criteria for Nursing Development Units

Salvage (1989) refers to the NDU as 'an umbrella description' which 'covers the work of health visitors, district nurses, midwives, mental health nurses and others as well as general hospital nurses' in a variety of settings. She adds 'What matters is not so much the name as the shared values and aspirations' (p. 25).

In 1994, Neal reported a total of 34 NDUs which had been endorsed by the King's Fund team. She describes the variety within NDUs as lying between two extremes of a scale. At one end of the scale are the 'nurture' units, which are at the beginning of their development. These units act primarily as a local resource for their parent organization and focus on the development and evaluation of practices. At the opposite end of the scale are the 'mature' units, 'which have already experienced considerable change and development and have moved their focus to research. Their contribution to the nursing profession and to health care is appreciable, making them a national resource'(p. 31).

Neal describes the more common variety of NDU as the one which falls between the two extremes of the scale. We place ourselves in this middle range: NDUs which 'undertake a balance of research, development and evaluation and whose sights are firmly fixed on becoming a local as well as a regional resource both in and outside nursing'(p. 31).

The following criteria have been used by the King's Fund to judge a unit's claim for NDU status. These criteria include commitment by both the unit and its 'parent' organization to the following:

- development of nursing
- clinical leadership
- organizational commitment
- staff participation
- staff development
- evaluation
- finance
- equal opportunities.

In preparing a case for King's Fund endorsement, the unit needs to demonstrate how each of these criteria will be interpreted and implemented. Key words in all of these criteria include: strategy, vision, team work, effective communication and commitment to change and evaluation. (All these criteria were considered in our proposal for NDU status.)

Our application to the King's Fund did not result in us receiving funding for our unit. There had been an overwhelming response to the Fund's call for proposals and in the end only six of them could be funded out of a total of 29 submissions. We did, however, receive endorsement from the King's Fund that we satisfied the criteria for acquiring NDU status. Our Achilles heel related to limited long-term organizational support from the health authority for the initiative. Organizational support requires a degree of stability which could not be guaranteed by our inner city health authority. At the time of our application the authority was undergoing management reorganization and major cutbacks associated with reduced spending on the health service. It is likely therefore that the King's Fund judges did not feel sufficiently confident in the health authority's ability to sustain long-term support and commitment to the project against a backdrop of far-reaching changes.

Despite us not securing the King's Fund money, our desire to develop and change was backed by a stronger confidence in ourselves and a belief in the value we could add to both patient care and nursing. Disappointed but undeterred, we decided to seek alternative sources of funding.

Recent history

Since the early days of the King's Fund initiative, further funding was provided by the Department of Health to support the expansion of NDUs (Vaughan, 1991). A national network was set up which encouraged NDU staff to share information and understanding about change processes. As members of that network we made visits to other units and gave talks as well as receiving visitors and telephone enquiries.

In 1994 two reports (Black, 1993; Turner-Shaw and Bosanquet, 1993) were published which gave accounts of the current state of NDUs. Medical opinion and patient views of the NDUs were curiously absent (Lorentzon, 1994). Like Lorentzon we were surprised by these gaps, given the demise of the Oxford Unit which was attributed to lack of medical support (Salvage, 1989) and the aim of NDUs to promote excellence in nursing care.

In our own case we were supported by the senior nurse managers of our hospital and the health authority which had a history of strong and committed nursing leadership. This began to change, however, following the 1990 health service reforms when health authorities as potential purchasers began to distance themselves from the provider units.

The medical support we received was mixed. Our consultants came from a variety of medical and surgical specialities and it was interesting that the haematologists shared a philosophy of care which was much closer to our own, which emphasized an holistic approach to patients. At the other end of the spectrum were the surgeons who tended to see patients in terms of conditions to be treated. They were uneasy about viewing us as equal partners in caring for patients whom they regarded as 'theirs'.

However, it was medical support, in the guise of the medical members of the Hospital Special Trustees, who finally funded our bid to become an NDU. Traditionally, the Special Trustees had only funded medical research carried out by hospital consultants and medical school staff. Our proposal was the first nursing project to obtain a grant from this fund. It was made possible by the development of a more open attitude on the part of medical academics towards nursing and PAMS (professions allied to medicine) research as a legitimate way forward for health services (as opposed to biomedical) research. The chair of the Clinical Research and Development committee, who worked closely with the Special Trustees in allocating funds, invited our senior nurse managers and nurse researcher to discuss possible ways forward for supporting nursing research. Our NDU proposal was submitted to and scrutinized by the Special Trustees. It was agreed that funding should be given for a three-year appointment of a nursing development facilitator to take the NDU proposal forward.

It was during the tenure of that appointment that the financial constraints imposed on the NHS began to hinder progress. Our ward was closed and amalgamated with a surgical unit. Attempts were made, however, to remain focused on the aims and objectives laid down in our NDU proposal as documented below.

The process of becoming a Nursing Development Unit

Our ward

Prior to the changes towards becoming a Nursing Development Unit in 1988, the ward had gained a positive reputation among both nursing and multidisciplinary staff within the hospital. This reputation was based on the ward being managed and run 'efficiently'. This efficiency seems to have been underpinned by a structured routine, attention to the neatness of the physical environment of the ward and a more traditional division of nursing duties among the nursing staff. The most senior nurse would be 'in charge', managing, for example, the 'ward round' or administration of medicines, rather than the care of an allocated group of patients. More junior staff were meanwhile assisting patients with personal care needs and undertaking a monitoring role, via the recording of routine blood pressures, temperature and pulse measurements.

The way nursing care was organized at this time seemed to relate most closely to patient allocation. Although the patient was the focus of the allocation, continuity of care was not a feature of it. The nursing staff appear to have been reluctant to explore continuity for two main reasons. First, to care for a wide variety of patients was considered to provide a greater opportunity for nurses to improve their knowledge and consequently different patients were allocated to each nurse every few days. Second, to care for the same patients on a continuous basis was considered by nurses to risk emotional involvement and therefore be a potential cause of stress. The potential benefit of continuity, for both nurses and patients, was not explored at this time. However, an Audit Commission Report (1991), entitled *The Virtue of Patients*, later confirmed the importance of continuity of care for patients, citing our unit as an example of good practice.

An investigation of the nursing as it existed before 1987, and the beginning of key changes, highlights several key features. The nursing staff provided not only a stable workforce (most of the nurses had worked on the unit between one and five years) but also a cohesive team. The nursing team not only cared for the patients and the physical environment of the ward, but also invested in their working relationships with each other and other professional groups, such as doctors, therapists and pharmacists.

The hospital context

As a backdrop to the changes on the ward, interest in developing clinical practice gathered momentum within the hospital itself. As described in our proposal, this centred on a nursing seminar led by Dr Susan Pembrey, who was heading up clinical nursing developments in Oxford Health Authority based at the Radcliffe Infirmary. Her presentation, in addition to a growing interest in the work of Alan Pearson in relation to primary nursing at Burford Community Hospital and Beeson ward in Oxford, began to fuel interest in a core group of nurses. These nurses then formed a team and primary nursing interest group, where a forum for exchanging ideas and supporting new ventures was provided. This activity, in addition to managerial support for research and development, helped to create a positive atmosphere towards changes within nursing.

This managerial support for research and development appeared to have been further reinforced, at this time, by recommendations originating from the then regional nurse. She requested that nurse managers focus on more holistic approaches to the organization of nursing care within their units, such as primary nursing.

Change and innovation

Introducing change in any area can be problematic. Every environment contains positive and negative forces which ideally need to be acknowledged, before the introduction of a change strategy. Our introduction of change in the early stages had no theoretical underpinning, and this no doubt accounted in part for some of the problems we encountered.

When applying retrospectively elements of change theory to our experience, certain aspects emerge as possible reasons why the changes introduced were ultimately positive ones. The driving or positive forces (Lewin, 1958) that were present within the unit included the stability of the workforce. The majority of the nursing staff had worked on the unit between one and five years, while the new senior staff nurse had previously worked alongside the ward sister and, therefore, was perhaps more readily accepted into the group. Staff also seemed comfortable with their levels of knowledge of how to care for the medical and nursing needs of patients admitted to the unit.

Their knowledge was underpinned by a good working relationship between themselves and other professional groups. Some members of the medical staff, but by no means all, were particularly supportive. They were vocal in their support both of the style of leadership and the management of the ward's nursing activity. The fact that the unit was considered to be running efficiently resulted in a greater willingness from both staff within and external to the unit to work through the period of instability and uncertainty which occurs when change is introduced.

Most of these issues, however, could have become counter or resisting forces (Lewin, 1958) when moving towards change, and it is now recognized that they potentially could have caused greater disharmony within the team. Additionally, change within the nursing profession was perhaps considered less favourable in 1987 than it is today. The climate of the time was less willing to accept new ideas and what would now be considered acceptable was greeted then as radical and a significant move from the security of tradition.

Initially, change occurred in a relatively unstructured and haphazard way. The new senior staff nurse, who later became the nursing development coordinator and was to be identified as the change agent (Wright, 1989), began to challenge the 'norm' of what was considered by many at the time as the adoption of a very critical stance on the way care was being organized. This approach may now be seen as using a more power-coercive strategy (Wright, 1989). While heated discussions and episodes of bad feelings pervaded the early stages of changing practice, staff slowly began to develop an understanding of the value of patient-centred care, and themselves question many nursing rituals.

While few actual changes to ward organization occurred in the first six months of the senior staff nurse (i.e. the change agent designate) being employed, this period of transition was fraught with disagreements as staff internalized new concepts of care at different speeds. Several members of staff developed hostile attitudes towards change and attempted to sabotage proposed new developments. For example, an agreement to devolve the management of patients to individual nurses had been made at one of many ward meetings. One of the key components of this change was that nurses would administer medications only for their group of allocated patients. This was one of the least contentious change issues, yet some staff continued with the old practice, whereby often the most senior nurses on duty administered medications to the whole ward with the attitude that this task had to be completed as quickly as possible. One member of staff considered the new ideology to be at such odds with the way she liked to provide care that she decided to resign.

On reflection, this approach to change was threatening to many staff and actually hindered progress. No agreements had been made and no framework had been identified to structure developments. A theory of change had not been considered to aid the transition, and two camps, led respectively by the ward sister and the change agent, each in danger of becoming polarized in their opinions of care, began to emerge. However, the unity and friendship that existed on the ward between the nursing staff meant that the emerging hostility remained focused on approaches to care, and did not seem to interfere with the social infrastructure that was a strong feature of the ward. The resistant staff attitudes began to change and a willingness to discuss plans for the introduction of primary nursing was accepted by the majority. This time a plan was devised to structure the introduction of primary nursing within a 12 month period.

It should be noted here that in addition to the support we received from the senior nursing management of the hospital, the willingness of the ward sister to allow her role on the ward to be challenged was, in retrospect, a significant factor in our progress. The ward sister initially faced a dilemma. She wanted to maintain her current status and style of management with which she felt secure, but could nevertheless see that the proposed changes were for the benefit of patients.

Creating the ward philosophy

Changing the focus of nursing towards the individual needs of the patient through primary nursing required more than a structural reorganization of the way care was delivered. It also required nurses to focus on the implementation of holistic nursing care. Primary nursing, according to Manthey (1980), is a method of organizing care but, like the nursing process, it is also said to encompass a philosophy of care (Hegyvary, 1982). In addition to the nursing knowledge and skills possessed by a group of care-givers, the most crucial determinant of how the patient is nursed lies in their philosophy of nursing (Pearson, 1983).

Within the ward at the time there was limited knowledge or experience of creating and writing a philosophy. Pervading the staff was a view that a philosophy is a paper exercise managers require, rather than something that can have an impact on the delivery of care. However, having arrived at the stage of agreeing to work towards the implementation of primary nursing, staff did agree to engage with the creation of a ward philosophy. Initially themes emerged that were agreed and these subsequently provided the structure for the written philosophy.

Integral to our philosophy were the concepts of the patient being cared for as an individual; that research should provide the basis for nursing practice while each person's opinion should be considered and respected; finally that the primary nurse should be provided with the best opportunity for high quality, autonomous practice.

The philosophy was felt to reflect the views of the staff until the first of many mergers with other wards. The philosophy was reviewed once only during the next five years, and that was as part of an article for a nursing journal, rather than any desire on the part of the staff. While a core of nurses remained within the ward for the five years of development, the requirement to amalgamate staff because of ward closures virtually on an annual basis, created a relatively high turnover of staff whose values about nursing covered a broad spectrum rather than forming a consensus. No doubt, part of the decision not to review the philosophy was an undisclosed feeling that the beliefs of staff would be radically different to those originally expressed, requiring coercion to get others to accept different values. This was indeed a dubious basis for a philosophy.

Primary nursing

Primary nursing is a method of care which has become a hallmark of many NDUs. As discussed by Abigail Masterson in Chapter 5 it grew exponentially from 'a mere whisper' in the 1970s to achieve quasi-statutory status as the 'named-nurse' component of *The Patient's Charter* (DoH, 1991). It is salutary to remember that one of the factors attributed to the growth in popularity of primary nursing is 'the new right-wing political and social values infiltrating Britain since 1979' which emphasized individual rather than collective goals (Finch 1991, p. 68). On the professional front, however, Pearson saw the development of primary nursing as a way of expanding the nurse's role to increase autonomy and accountability and ultimately better patient care.

The successful implementation of primary nursing involves managing a complex change process by altering the way nurses think about nursing, how they practice nursing, and how nursing is organized (Johns, 1991). The framework adapted for organizing and leading our change process was based on the account by Pearson in his book entitled *The Clinical Nursing Unit* (1983) and other accounts of activities in the Burford Community Hospital and the Radcliffe Infirmary's Beeson ward.

Our starting point for the introduction of primary nursing was the education of staff both about primary nursing and holistic care. Suggested reading was provided and ideas and issues discussed at ward meetings. A decision on how to start, however, was not easily clarified. We were fortunate at this point to receive assistance from the senior nurse for research and development who wished to maintain clinical contact in an area where she had previously undertaken research. It was with her guidance that primary nursing became the established organization of nursing care.

Evaluation and quality

While we did not have a lot of experience and knowledge of the change process, we realized that in order to evaluate the effectiveness of our proposed change, it seemed sensible to undertake a measurement of the quality of care before and after the introduction of primary nursing.

The initial assessment using QualPacs (Wandelt and Ager, 1974) allowed us to set a baseline for later evaluation of the effects of primary nursing on patient care. It allowed us to gain some experience in quality measurement tools and allowed us to focus on areas of care which required further improvement. It also gave encouragement and confidence to the ward team by highlighting the areas of nursing care which were shown to be above average. While accepting the limitations of QualPacs however, we were able to interpret the findings by using the observational feedback as well as the actual score.

One value of QualPacs is that it provides the opportunity for peer review and most staff who had worked on the unit for more than a year were trained in the use of this tool. Staff feedback was very positive. The main benefit noted was that it gave nurses a rare opportunity to sit and observe care for a period of time and in so doing enabled them to reflect on their own practice.

It needs to be said that nurses can often feel uncomfortable, even threatened, by the assessment of quality and observation of their care on the ward. The reason why the use of QualPacs was effective in our case was, we believe, because it was not enforced in a top–down approach, and the results were at that stage for our interpretation only. We felt comfortable assessing care because it was our collective decision to do so.

Irrespective of these factors, being audited by an experienced external assessor created an additional pressure in case our belief that we provided a good level of service was not reflected in the results. Repeated peer review removed this concern and we were eager to be made aware of aspects of care that required further improvements.

The focus in the 1990s has changed to one of valuing outcome indicators with the main focus being cost-effectiveness. While this has a place in nursing, there is a danger of relying solely on this approach, to the detriment of ignoring other valuable areas of quality such as the process.

Care-planning as a key outcome

The quality of care plans improved significantly throughout the early stages of development on the ward. The emphasis changed from care-planning being little more than a 'necessary evil' required legally as part of the nursing process, to a valuable working document, which informed practice and involved patients in planning care.

Like Helen Mann (see Chapter 8) we felt that written explicit care plans as part of documentation were an essential vehicle to providing detailed information on patient needs and to support what was said verbally. A lot of time and energy was channelled into educating staff on the basic principles of care-planning, focusing on four fundamental principles. All care plans were to be:

1   patient-focused and patient-worded
2   have realistic, measurable and achievable goals
3   written, when possible, with the patient
4   constantly reviewed.

The transition was, however, not smooth for many staff who had received little more than a cursory glance at care-planning during their nurse training and therefore never appreciated the benefits of a comprehensive plan. However, once familiar with utilizing the fundamental principles, staff were able to identify many advantages. Some of the advantages identified included a minimal chance of forgetting small issues relating to the patient, such as 'PC prefers bed covers not to be tucked in as this increases itching to feet'; phrasing problems became easier as they were based on what the patient said, rather than how the nurse described them; the time spent with patients in a therapeutic way was increased; writing helped to focus thinking and focused thinking helped to improve practice. Finally, a sentiment shared by all the nurses who had worked on the unit was the difficulties they encountered when they moved to environments where patients did not have care plans that met our criteria.

Computerized care plans

Whether many of our fundamental principles survive the emergence of computer systems for developing care plans remains debatable. The opportunity for nurses to involve patients in the care-planning process and produce jargon-free text is increasingly difficult because of the limitations inherent in software packages. This becomes virtually impossible when, as is often the case, there is only one fixed computer terminal per ward. The challenge of focusing thinking before writing individual plans of care has also been eroded because a catalogue of problems exists covering the requested topic area on the computer for nurses to access. The essential component of individuality is missing. Inevitably, the true benefits of manual care-planning to enhance patient care are lost. When care-planning is computerized it becomes devalued as little more than a nursing ritual.

A study of district nurses illustrated the restrictions imposed by computerized information systems on interpreting, developing and documenting their work. The researchers reported that the nurses were doubtful that the codes and categories being developed to document their work were sufficiently sensitive to reflect the holistic nature of their activities (Smith, Towers and Mackintosh, 1993). The following vignette illustrates this point. On return from her patient visits, a new staff member experienced initial difficulty in completing the computer activity record. As she began inputting her activities she soon encountered difficulties in selecting the appropriate categories and codes. The administration of injections, for example, was classified under 'technical procedures' but the nurse also wanted to include talking to patients as part of this activity. On the computer record, 'talking' featured under the heading 'support codes' if it had served a specific function of giving 'advice/support'. When 'talking' took place as part of a more general social interaction, then no code existed.

The researchers also reported that participant observation confirmed the limitations of the system in capturing the personalization of nursing care received by patients.

NDUs and the health care market

It is worth noting that when seeking funding in the present climate, nurses face a different set of challenges than in the early days of the King's Fund initiative. The language and intent of the proposal must place greater emphasis on making explicit what might have previously been taken for granted in a pre-market NHS. With the introduction of the internal market and purchasers and providers, funding proposals need to adopt the terminology and language of business plans based on marketability and cost. Proposals for nursing innovations need to identify the outcomes of nursing innovations in terms of benefits and costs. In other words, the proposer needs to convince purchasers that what they would get from setting up a contract with an NDU would both ensure quality and save money.

Barbie Vaughan, Jane Salvage's successor as Director of the King's Fund nursing development programme, had no doubt that NDUs offered three critical outcome benefits which were of interest to both purchasers and providers. First, they served as 'a "laboratory" for the development of practice'. Second they acted as a 'resource for teaching and consultancy' and third, they provided 'a demonstration site for good practice' (Vaughan, 1992, p. 28).

Improving and developing practice, therefore, could be described as 'value added nursing' which is further demonstrated by a research approach to practice. When practice is backed up by research, the purchaser has proof of its 'marketability'. The acceptance of a particular research approach, however, depends on the purchaser's understanding of research. It may be that providers are obliged to communicate in a way that is prechosen, for example, through presenting evidence from clinical trials/randomized controlled trials as defined by the NHS R&D strategy rather than using qualitative means such as reflective practice and story-telling. Furthermore, the introduction of the market and its associated language potentially divides practitioners by encouraging competition at the expense of collaboration.

The potential divisiveness of the market is illustrated by Mangan (1992) who argues that:

> Commercially, the prestige that comes from having NDU status can be highly marketable in today's health service. Units striving to compete for 'business' against other provider units could be forgiven for stressing that the quality of their nursing service has been recognised and that their practice is based on providing research-based nursing at the highest level.(p. 29)

Mason (1994) further suggests that:

> NDU values of equality, democracy, esteem-building and personal growth are relevant to the business philosophy of the NHS.

With regards to cost-effectiveness she concludes that:

> NDUs are already in the lead since for over ten years their nurses first started to critically evaluate their practice, instigate change, and monitor outcomes. For these reasons, NDUs are surely in a strong position to argue a case to purchasers in favour of their further development. (p. 36)

The setting up of NDUs is not without controversy. Some critics believe their establishment breeds élitism and rifts between nurses who are members of NDUs and those who are not. Their presence may also suggest that innovative practice and high standards are not possible elsewhere. Neal's (1994) characterization of NDUs helps to counter these criticisms by showing that there is a wide variety of activity across the two extremes of 'nurture' and 'mature' units. However, as our own experience shows, NDUs cannot happen without the commitment of the parent organization to resources, including the employment of staff not only in adequate numbers but also with sufficient clinical expertise to work as an expert nurse, innovator and team-player.

Speaking the language of new management was not something we as practising nurses were familiar with. Therefore the element of risk-taking which is a feature of many advances in nursing was less acceptable without quantifiable evidence as a reason for introducing a change. Taking unsubstantiated risks was less well tolerated by non-nurse managers who were not used to dealing with intuitive requests. This is why we have dedicated the next section of the chapter to exploring the generation of knowledge through practice as a form of evidence-based research which can be used as a way of substantiating intuition.

Generating knowledge

The creation of new knowledge was not undertaken as an end in itself or as a conscious process, although we were aware of our desire to contribute to the progression of nursing practice. We also felt a responsibility to use research evidence in our care-planning and decision-making. The generation of new knowledge occurred as a natural process.

The process of change leading up to the implementation of primary nursing and the continued progress made during that time inevitably brought about a new philosophy and culture on the ward in which nurses had a much more questioning approach. The reasons for current practice were not taken for granted, nor was it accepted that there was only one way of doing things. Accepted principles were not necessarily accepted as the best.

Nurses were encouraged to pursue an area of interest and build up a portfolio of articles and research reports, thus providing a written as well as a personal source of knowledge and expertise to colleagues. Written accounts in several forms, whether they were literature reviews, care plans, 'standards', journal articles or reports, while having many functions, served as a way of codifying, formalizing and legitimizing forms of empirical knowledge.

Empirical knowledge and its association with experimental method could be easily identified from these accounts because of its relationship to a factual and scientific knowledge-base but also to what could be tangibly gained and learned through experience. Similarities between clinical observations and experimentation can be noted. Take, for example, the condition of hyperpyrexia. A nurse could be expected to understand its likely cause in a particular patient, know what signs to look for, what action to take, as well as the effect of the action taken. She would therefore be looking for cause and effect: the cause of the hyperpyrexia in the first place; the effects it was having on the patient; the intervention required to lower body temperature and the signs which indicated its effectiveness.

Written accounts also existed as a form of evidence to ourselves and our managers, that our knowledge was increasing. This was important to us for documenting both the process and effects of change in the unit. Staff were encouraged to write and share information with staff and patients and also with a wider audience through publication. Like Helen Mann in Chapter 8, we saw our care plans and reports as a means of accruing evidence about our everyday practice.

As Colleen Wedderburn Tate indicated in Chapter 2, knowledge is often not accredited unless it is written down or can be ascribed to an 'expert'. In the scientific and medical world, empirical knowledge is often viewed as the only legitimate form of knowledge. While talking and writing about our practice, we began to recognize another form of knowledge which may go unrecognized and therefore remain invisible. This is intuitive knowledge and although in our experience it is undoubtedly an important aspect of nurses' practice, it is a form that remains hard to identify and define.

While both empirical and intuitive forms of knowledge are referred to in this chapter, we would like to argue the presence of another even less tangible form of knowledge. Differences in quality of care, the way care is carried out, ward philosophies and perhaps even ward cultures may be explained by the presence of this particular knowledge form.

In taking this discussion further, we refer to the work of Carper (1978) who identifies four fundamental patterns of knowing:

1   empirics, the science of nursing
2   aesthetics, the art of nursing
3   the component of a personal knowledge in nursing
4   ethics, the component of moral knowledge in nursing.

The following vignette illustrating an example of care will be used to explore different aspects of knowledge by providing an analysis using Carper's framework. The aim of such an analysis is, however, not to identify the extent and range of nurses' knowledge, but to address the meanings and value accorded to more implicit kinds of knowledge within nursing.

This vignette is a summary of a case study described by Jan Savage (1995) in her book on *Nursing Intimacy* (pp. 55–7). The case study refers to the relationship between a primary nurse 'Jane' and an elderly patient 'Lee' whom she had nursed for approximately three years. The patient had known that he had cholangiocarcinoma before he and Jane first met. A metal stent had been inserted for the purpose of relieving a blockage of the bile system. Lee's frequent admissions to hospital were for the purpose of maintaining the patency of the stent. In terms of nursing needs, Lee required very little physical care. But he and Jane spent considerable time talking to and finding out about each other. Lee spoke at length about his life in China and his family.

When Lee was hospitalized for what was to be his last admission, Jane realized immediately that this time 'it was different' even though treatment proceeded in the usual manner. Lee slowly began to realize he would not recover. He would cry 'for no particular reason it seemed' but only in Jane's presence. Her response was to 'just sit and hold his hand, for ages really'. Eventually Lee was referred for an ultrasound scan which showed that 'there was little more that could be done for him'.

We quote the following extracts in full because of their explanatory power in terms of understanding a form of knowledge that is intangible and goes beyond empirical and even intuitive forms.

When Lee returned to the ward following the ultrasound, Jane recalled:

> the pharmacist was just by his bed and he said to her, 'Oh, they've told me they can't do any more'; he was quite matter of fact about it. And then the pharmacist said later that she'd been struck by the fact that when I came over to him, he'd instantly burst into tears and told me the same thing. She moved away quite tactfully, and I pulled the curtain round and spent quite a lot of time with him. But she told me later she realized then what a difference in the relationship there was between her and him and myself and him'.

The quality of Jane's relationship with Lee also allowed her to challenge the medical team's opinion that he was denying the reality of the situation. Rather, her knowledge of Lee permitted Jane to say 'to the doctors that I felt he had accepted it . . . he might be denying it a little bit . . . it's only natural to want to keep on living'. He told Jane that although he didn't want to die he recognized 'I'm old, my body's old and I can't live like this.'

On reflecting on their relationship, after Lee died, Jane supposed:

> It made me realize how much importance [patients] do attach to a person, or two or three people they've known for quite a long time. And the fact that you can communicate without . . . that you can cut the formalities really . . . *that you can communicate at a different level* . . . it made me ask a lot of questions about the way you look after somebody; you can't just write it in the care plan as something you should do. (Researcher's emphasis)

From this short case study we can identify through Carper's (1978) framework that the nurse was drawing on different elements of knowledge in her care of the patient. Empathy is described by Carper as 'the capacity for participating in or vicariously experiencing another's feelings' (p. 219) and is a key component of her aesthetic pattern of knowing. It is clear that the nurse in the above example was drawing on her 'aesthetic' knowledge in her support and comfort of Lee. The fourth type of knowledge identified by Carper is that associated with moral decision-making and ethics. The nurse may also have been drawing on her 'ethical' knowledge in her intervention with the doctors in discussing Lee's reaction to the results of his ultrasound. She was also undoubtedly using her 'personal knowledge' throughout all her interactions with Lee. This pattern of knowing categorized by Carper is probably the most difficult to understand and relate to patient care. It is concerned with the 'knowing, encountering and actualizing' of the concrete, individual self. One does not know *about* the self; one strives simply to *know* the self. This knowing is a standing in relation to another human being and confronting that human being as a person (p. 220). It is about the personal knowledge unique to each individual and about the use of 'self' in our relationship with others.

However, we think there may be another element or form of knowledge which is not explained by Carper's model and of which we were unaware at the time. It is only now through reflective analyses and grappling with the concept of intuitive knowledge that we realize that another sort of knowledge exists and are able to make it explicit and therefore visible. This additional type of knowledge is important because if recognized it can help us learn about aspects of nursing which are very difficult to identify, for example, what care can be comprised of and what it can mean. So is it necessary and is it even possible to articulate what this new element of knowledge is about? If it can't be identified and spoken about, then it can't be learned from or used to give value to nursing.

We suggest 'knowing the person', and by this we mean having an in-depth knowledge of the patient as a person, which can be developed further over time, is another type of knowledge which does not seem to be explained within Carper's model. Neither can it be situated entirely within the concept of intuitive knowledge. But it is more about a 'special' relationship with a patient, on a particular ward. It is more than knowing *about* the person, but about *knowing* the person. This sounds familiar in the light of Carper's definition of personal knowing, but although 'knowing the person' may well overlap to a greater or lesser extent with many other types of knowledge, we believe it is also something extra which adds another dimension to care-giving.

Intuitive knowledge is described by Tanner (1989) as judgement without rationale; it is about doing something without conscious reasoning. It is acknowledged that expert practitioners will often use intuitive knowledge and they are able to do this because of their level of experience and knowledge. Benner (1984) in her now classic text *From Novice to Expert* states:

> A wealth of untapped knowledge is embedded in the practices and the 'know-how' of expert nurse clinicians, but this knowledge will not expand or fully develop unless nurses systematically record what they learn from their own experience. Clinical expertise has not been adequately described or compensated in nursing, and the lag in description contributes to the lag in recognition and reward. (p. 11)

Benner's descriptions of untapped knowledge embedded in the practices and the 'know-how' of experts is, for us, describing the process associated with the acquisition of 'intuitive' knowledge.

However, while 'experience is a requisite for expertise' (Benner, 1984, p. 3) and decision-making as well as problem-solving becomes increasingly more skilful and sophisticated as nurses progress from novice to expert, we must also recognize that intuitive knowledge may sometimes be displayed by the most junior members of the ward team, be they student nurses or health care assistants. We suggest that this may be possible not through experience, but through their special knowledge of or relationship with a patient. Smith (1992) in her book *The Emotional Labour of Nursing* which includes her analysis of the socialization of student nurses, describes third-year students' views of first years who had an 'uncanny way of knowing their patients' which the third-years recognized they had lost (p. 113).

It is a paradox that nurses' socialization into their profession can cause them to lose skills which can make a real difference to patients and the care given to them. Smith (1992) also describes how some student nurses challenged this socialization, broke away from the hierarchy and talked about patients as real people (see pages 107–110).

We believed that knowing the person was a fundamental part of caring for them. We also recognized the individuality of staff as well as patients. As individuals, nurses get to know different things about their patients, come to know them in different ways and relate to them all differently. This applies equally whatever level the nurse is at. The most junior members of the ward team were often unable to express their views or feelings about a patient in detail, or by using specific terminology, and what they articulated verbally couldn't necessarily be measured or written down. However, our belief in their knowledge of the patient meant that we valued what they had to say and took it seriously. Their knowledge was acquired by caring for their patients throughout their admission and by working in an environment where great importance was attached to talking to patients and where nurses were encouraged to communicate their concerns freely.

We want to emphasize, though, that what we are describing in terms of nurses' special knowledge is not unique to the environment of a Nursing Development Unit, but can occur wherever nursing takes place and where patients are the focus of all care. However, a Nursing Development Unit can provide a creative environment in which nurses are free to introduce innovations and develop nursing practice, as highlighted by Black (1992).

As stated earlier, we held a strong belief that the most experienced nurses should be providing direct patient care and providing a role model to colleagues. This meant that we worked closely *with* students, junior qualified staff and health care assistants rather than delegate separate activities to them and work apart. As a result nurses were not isolated from each other, the cohesiveness of the ward team was strengthened and patient care was not fragmented.

Where NDUs might differ from a regular hospital ward might be in the opportunity they offer to recognize the different ways of knowing in nursing practice. We compare describing the intangible elements of knowing to wiping up spilt mercury from a broken thermometer. The mercury, like the element of knowing we are trying to describe, defies attempts to capture or contain it, fragmenting into a myriad of elusive droplets. We maintain that as nurses it is important to accept that elements of our knowledge may be elusive but it is still important to acknowledge their presence.

Research and development

The type of research carried out on NDUs tends to emphasize the development aspects of R&D. The staff on our unit were no exception. We needed to see research as accessible and at a level at which we could underpin practice. In this respect, the application and generation of research has an obvious relationship with the generation of knowledge.

For a lot of nurses there is a sense that research exists in 'ivory towers'; that it is carried out only by those in academic departments and that it is devoid of meaning for the clinical practitioner. We were anxious to dispel these attitudes and believed that while not all nurses are or should be researchers, they should be comfortable accessing up-to-date research findings, appraising them and incorporating them into the care they plan and provide.

A research interest group provided a forum in which to discuss published articles with the purpose of demystifying research in general and helping to promote research-mindedness among staff. All nurses on the ward were involved, including health care assistants. Everyone was encouraged to share their interests and involvement in research whatever the level, from those who had carried out literature searches to others who had expertise in specific research methods and had instigated original studies.

Thus to instinctively identify the use of research as an essential aspect of nursing care became part of our nursing culture. In other words, we asked questions about our practice that could only be answered by looking at the findings of appropriate research studies which had been carried out. Where it seemed no answers existed, we had to carry out small-scale research studies ourselves. The topics of our studies included bedside handovers, mixed-sex wards and temperature-taking. These small-scale studies were both necessary and helpful for evaluating the process and outcome of standard-setting.

Staff also benefited from the presence on the unit of outside academic researchers involved in large-scale studies who approached us wishing to use the ward as a study area. Their interest in our work and their integration into the ward team went a long way towards demystifying the research process for many of us and also provided us with a willing source of expert knowledge into which we could tap. Their research interests also coincided with a number of the topics we had identified in our King's Fund proposal as being in need of investigation.

The unit environment encouraged people to acquire research expertise and funding. Two members of staff undertook the ENB's 870 course, *An Introduction to the Understanding and Application of Research*. One of them, a primary nurse, obtained Regional Health Authority monies to fund a study on the perceptions of associate nurses working within the unit.

A potential drawback of a research friendly environment is that patients and staff will become 'over-researched'. We were careful to make sure that the research carried out on the unit coincided with our R&D plans. Furthermore we wanted to ensure that any research carried out would make a positive contribution to the functioning of the unit, rather than simply adding to our workload.

In summary, the research carried out on the unit either by ourselves or others demonstrated the importance of practice in informing research questions and processes, as well as practice and the generation of knowledge as a form of research.

Conclusion

The time when we submitted our King's Fund proposal was a time of great optimism when we believed nursing had undergone 'a great shift' from subservience to power. In concluding this chapter we would like to reflect on that statement.

We still believe that nurses have the potential to be powerful, to develop and control changes within their profession and to be more directive in the definition of their own role. For example, if nurses could sell the value of nursing and the potential for quality provision as well as cost-savings to both patients and institutions, a sufficient shift in the locus of control and power may occur for nurses to take a more active lead in decision-making about changes at ward, organizational and national levels.

As has been discussed elsewhere in this book, nursing and nurses as a group are often marginalised. NDUs are one way of bringing nursing to the fore. They provide a forum in which to demonstrate and explore the value of nursing and the difference they are able to make in terms of patient care. The establishment of NDUs was a rare opportunity whereby money was made available solely for nursing developments and this demonstrated that nursing was valued. The subsequent closure of many NDUs once external funding was no longer available has been indicative of a lack of managerial support, and the failure to sustain this initiative into the 1990s has yet again reinforced a view of nursing as a marginalized profession.

Forces allowing the closure of NDUs exist within the current climate especially since organizational restructuring and the emergence of the internal market. Although we recognize that the marketplace may create opportunities for recognizing the value of NDUs and nursing, this was not borne out by our own experience. Organizational changes in the management structure of our hospital and its transfer to Trust status meant many profound changes throughout the hospital. It marked the beginning of a long period of uncertainty and a feeling of insecurity and instability among nurses.

We realize in retrospect that changes within the hospital marked a period of great transition during which we felt our priorities refocused on survival strategies rather than developments. This was not because as a group we couldn't respond and adapt to change; nor was it because primary nursing can only function in one sort of setting. But using an analogy to illustrate our point, it is rather like asking if a house would still stand if its foundations were removed and not replaced with a different but equally secure base.

There was a feeling of resentment, anger and frustration at the lack of support for our endeavours and the open opposition to the concept of an NDU. We cannot emphasize enough the destructive effect this had on the ward team. Not having a secure environment meant that we were limited in our ability to try out new ideas, be creative and continue to challenge the accepted 'norm'. Any new ideas had now to be presented to non-nurses as a viable proposition. A convincing argument would have to be prepared in advance. This was very different to the previous system when ward-level nurses could approach a nurse manger who would then intercede on their behalf with those further up the management line and help explain and support changes.

We have written this chapter to give support to others who might have gone, or be going through, similar situations. We also show that although our NDU no longer exists as we have described it in this chapter, the people who were influenced by it, both patients and nurses, still do. The fact that we have now documented our experiences in these pages means that the ideas, processes and outcomes created during our time of working on an NDU have been recorded as evidence. We were all changed by our experiences. One of our colleagues summed up this change during a recent focus-group discussion of former NDU staff as part of a research project. We would like to conclude with her testimony:

> I think the experience I've had working over six years in practice with the group of us here has given me the enthusiasm for doing the work I do now to try and make it as good as I can. And I know it can be done, and it keeps me going and striving for the best.

In the new climate promised by the recent change in government we are again optimistic that opportunities will open up to support nurses to strive for the best, to enable 'a great shift' from subservience to power.

Acknowledgement

We would like to thank Shelagh Sparrow for permission to quote from her unpublished dissertation.

References

Audit Commission Report (1991) *The Virtue of Patients: Making Best Use of Ward Nursing Resources.* HMSO, London.

Benner P (1984) *From Novice to Expert,* Addison-Wesley, Thousand Oaks.

Black G (1992) *Work in Progress: an Overview.* Kings Fund Centre, London.

Black M (1993) *Nursing Development Units: The Growth of Tameside Nursing Development Unit: An exploration of Perceived Changes in Nursing Practice over a 10-Year Period.* King's Fund Centre, London.

Carper B A (1978) Fundamental patterns of knowing in nursing. *Advances in Nursing Science,* 1(1): 13–23.

Department of Health (1991) *The Patient's Charter.* HMSO, London.

Finch M (1991) The steady advance of a revolution. *Nursing Times* 87 (17): 67–8.

Hegyvary S T (1982) *The Change to Primary Nursing: A Cross-cultural View of Professional Practice.* C V Mosby, St Louis.

Johns C (1991) Introducing and managing change – the move to primary nursing. In Ersser S and Tutton E (eds) *Primary Nursing in Perspective.* Scutari Press, Harrow.

Lewin K (1958) Group decision and social change. In Maccoby E (ed.) *Readings in Social Psychology.* Holt, Rinehart & Winston, New York.

Lorentzon M (1994) Nursing development units: professionalization strategy for nurses, cheap service option or genuine improvement in patient care. *Journal of Advanced Nursing* (guest editorial) 19: 835–36.

Mangan P (1992) Protecting the species. *Nursing Times* 88 (31): 28–9.

Manthey M (1980) A theoretical framework for primary nursing. *Journal of Nursing Administration* 10 (6): 11–15.

Mason C (1994) NDUs: can they fit in a market-led service? *Nursing Standard* 9(1) 34–6.

Maxwell-Hudson C (1987) *The Complete Book of Massage*. Random House, London.

Merleau-Ponty M (1962) *The Phenomenology of Perception*. Routledge & Kegan Paul, London.

Neal K (1994) The function and aims of nursing development units. *Nursing Times* 90 (41): 31–3

Pearson A (1983) *The Clinical Nursing Unit*. Heinemann Medical Books, London.

Salvage J (1989) *Nursing developments*. *Nursing Standard* 22 (3): 25–8

Savage J (1995) *Nursing Intimacy: An Ethnographic Approach to Nurse–Patient Interaction*. Scutari Press, London.

Smith P (1992) *The Emotional Labour of Nursing: How Nurses Care*. Macmillan, Basingstoke.

Smith P, Towers B and Mackintosh M (1993) Implications of the new NHS contracting system for the district nursing service in one health authority: a pilot study. *Journal of International Care* 7(2): 115–124.

Tanner C A (1989) Using knowledge in clinical judgement. In Tanner C A and Lindeman C (eds) *Using Nursing Research*. National League for Nursing, New York.

Turner-Shaw B and Bosanquet N (1993) *Nursing Development Units: A Way to Develop Nurses and Nursing*. King's Fund Centre, London.

Vaughan B (1991) A new hand on the tiller. *Nursing Standard* 6 (11): 18–19.

Vaughan B (1992) The pursuit of excellence. *Nursing Times* 88 (31): 26–8.

Wandelt M and Ager J (1974) *Quality Patient Care Scale*. Appleton, Century, Crofts, Nowark.

Wright S (1989) *Changing Nursing Practice*. Edward Arnold, London.

10

Epilogue:
setting new research agendas

Angie Cotter and Pam Smith

In this chapter the authors draw on the preceding book chapters to show how the nursing research enterprise is in transition. A case is made for redefining research as a dynamic, ongoing process shaped by practice. The chapter draws out the main themes from the preceding chapters and makes further inferences for future research. Should, for example, nursing develop its own unique methodology or incorporate a variety of paradigms and approaches? Parallels are also drawn between psychotherapy and the research process. In conclusion, the authors speculate on a nursing and health care research agenda for the millennium.

Introduction

In this chapter we draw on the preceding book chapters to show how the research enterprise within nursing is in transition. We make a case for redefining research as a dynamic, ongoing process shaped by practice. We also show how research is a constellation of theories, knowledge, methodologies and practice that is shaped by history, society and biography. The chapter is divided into two sections. The first section draws out the main themes from the preceding chapters and makes further inferences from them. Key themes are identified with potential for moving the research agenda towards the millennium. The second section grew out of a chance conversation between the authors. We followed this up with several joint discussion and writing sessions. The process of producing the chapter represents a serendipitous collaboration which we experienced as being a more fruitful way of speculating on the issues facing nursing and health care research as we move into the twenty-first century.

The nursing and health care context

The introduction of the market economy into health care has affected nursing in ways we may only just be beginning to appreciate. The separation of purchasers and providers with the development of contracting relationships has meant a focus on cost-consciousness, which in turn means that nursing has had to attempt to quantify its products. Additionally the paperwork has increased with the need to keep accounts. These and other major influences on the development of nursing and nursing research are considered by Maureen Lahiff, Maria Lorentzon and Abigail Masterson in Chapters 3, 4 and 5 respectively.

The effects of the market on health care have been observed by a number of researchers including Traynor and Wade (1994) in their study about nurses' morale in three NHS Trusts. One quote from a nurse is illustrative: 'The ... trust is a business, managers are no longer concerned about employees as people while the welfare of clients comes secondary to saving money' (p. 42).

The introduction of informatics such as the computerization of records and the compilation of databases on cost and clinical effective care is also linked to the apparent commercialization of health care. Maria Lorentzon refers to the Cochrane and York centres, which have been set up to conduct systematic reviews and disseminate findings throughout the NHS. These changes require nurses and midwives to learn new skills, in an area which many may perceive as peripheral rather than central to their work. Computerization changes the communication patterns between nurses and other members of the health care team. In particular, written and verbal forms of communication may be changed by the introduction of computerized records as suggested by Anne Jones and Olwyn Bamford in Chapter 9. On the positive side, the compilation of databases about evidence-based treatments and organization provides up-to-date information to which nurses and users can have access. The danger here, as Colleen Wedderburn Tate points out in Chapter 2, is that health professionals and commissioners may make decisions about clinical care based on randomized controlled trials, which may overlook some of the complexities and uniqueness of each situation. The use of telemedicine and the internet also has the potential to distance the patient's individual experience even further from the health care professional.

Another trend related to the concept of the internal market is the emphasis on consumerism which has had a double-edged effect. The positive side is that there is now a legitimate focus on empowering health care users and involving them in their care, as well as the potential, as Colleen Wedderburn Tate suggests, for putting neglected and marginalized groups on the agenda. The downside is that nurses, unless they themselves become empowered, may experience the emphasis of involving users and carers as an additional pressure because of a lack of time and skill. Equally patients may conceptualize a chosen interest, knowing how to make that choice and to select criteria against which to measure their care (Neuberger, 1993).

At the time of writing a new Labour government has recently been elected. Their manifesto pledges include a re-examination and reform of the internal market. While the form of the internal market may change, it is unlikely that the associated issues outlined above will disappear.

Within nursing itself, the UKCC's (1992) *The Scope of Professional Practice* has opened the door to greater flexibility in the nursing role and the potential to become an advanced practitioner. Together with the moves towards reducing junior doctors' hours, this has resulted in conflicts for nurses at grass-roots level between developing technical skills and sustaining emotional care of the patient, and of each other, as the following quotation from a survey conducted in the USA illustrates:

> [nurses] no longer have time for a caring attitude. Cost containment means technical skills take precedence over teaching, psychological support and frequent turning and positioning. (Collins, 1988)

Additionally, in certain areas, notably community nursing, the traditional nursing work of personal care has been downloaded to the Home Care division of Social Services Departments (Smith *et al.*, 1996; Wade, 1996). Further, within continuing care, Social Services Departments are now funding most nursing home care which would seem to imply that continuing care nursing is not regarded as health care.

While the definitions of nursing work may be shifting, the doctor–nurse relationship remains a crucial factor to consider in the context of nursing. Maureen Lahiff and Abigail Masterson explore this factor in their respective chapters. In particular Maureen explores the gender dimension in health care generally, drawing on the early experiences of women entering medicine. She concludes that these gender divisions within health care are still in operation and result in ongoing tensions between doctors and nurses in relation to power, autonomy and control. Abigail cites Elliot's (1989) argument that nursing is systematically silenced at all levels and in all types of communication. The pragmatics of nursing discourse, it is suggested, are not considered official or noteworthy by the 'male' world of medicine and health care finance. The language of medicine remains the 'official' language of health care.

Nursing research

Moving to the context of nursing research, several authors lament the resultant lack of nurses on influential R&D committees. The Culyer Report (DoH, 1994) offers both an opportunity and a challenge for nursing. One set of recommendations within the Report was specifically aimed at improving the chances of 'Cinderella' settings and disciplines to secure research funding. The challenge, as Maria Lorentzon suggests in Chapter 4, comes from the fact that no direct reference to nursing is made in the report. Therefore, nurses with R&D remits in NHS Trusts must be proactive to ensure their research priorities are represented.

This general situation partly explains why certain topics and methodologies get funded over and against those which are seen to be of marginal interest as highlighted by Maureen Lahiff, Trudi James and Dawn Whittaker. Additionally, Gosia Brykczyńska cites Feyerabend's view that professionals can use research to reinforce a blinkered approach to their discipline which can lead to 'professionalized incompetence'. Several authors imply that nursing is attempting through scholarly endeavour to attain the credentials which, it is argued, will give nurses greater influence in the multidisciplinary arena. Ironically, these endeavours move nurses away from the bedside and could be seen therefore to reinforce Feyerabend's notion of 'professionalized incompetence'. This may explain, therefore, the historical and current ambivalence of nursing leaders towards academic nursing, noted by Maureen Lahiff.

In this context it is interesting to reflect on the origins of research as a 'gentleman's occupation', available to a privileged élite with private means, as characterised by the Oxbridge don. Margaret Wertheim's (1995) history of the development of modern physics, traditionally regarded as the benchmark by which present-day science and research is judged, shows how the discipline grew from the close alliance between religion, the Catholic Church and male supremacy. The first European universities, set up to educate the clergy, excluded women, and it was 1882 before fellows of Oxford and Cambridge were allowed to marry.

The history of the institutionalized male academic, whose sole activity was the pursuit of scholarship, may have current vestiges in the fact that undertaking research is costly. The fees required to undertake masters and doctoral studies are expensive and as sources of public funding dry up, there is an increase in the number of students who are self-financing. Cost-conscious health service managers also pose the question whether researchers should pay an institution for the participants' time (especially if they are practitioners) to take part in research. Nursing and social work training still serves to limit reflection and thinking time in favour of 'doing' (take for example Project 2000's emphasis on the 'knowledgeable *doer*' rather than thinker).

On the other hand, theoretical disciplines such as physics may be too abstract. Wertheim (1995) is critical of current priorities within physics, for example, which she describes as the pursuit of a 'Theory of Everything' unconnected with reality. She concludes: 'No knowledge, for its own sake is worth this price . . . we need a physics that is more centred on human needs and concerns . . . we must be involved in deciding . . . what purposes we want [physics] to serve.'

The practitioners' views in Chapters 8 and 9 can be set against a theory of science which derives knowledge from experimentation divorced from the 'real' world. For example, Anne Jones and Olwyn Bamford accept the legitimacy of intuitive knowledge in their experience. Helen Mann's chapter shows how a reflective research-based approach to frontline care can be used to recognize the nursing skills necessary in the development of a new specialist role. These chapters are of particular relevance when considering the development of models for advanced practice.

Forms of knowledge, which sit uneasily with the traditional scientific view, such as 'magic' and intuition, stand even less chance of receiving serious consideration. However, it is useful to be reminded by Wertheim (1995) that historically the differences between science and magic were not so clearly demarcated.

In a similiar vein, Colleen Wedderburn Tate critiques how the Western positivist perspective defines what counts as knowledge, denigrating the wisdom and insight of those without academic qualifications and training. This dominance affects the assessment of what counts as evidence which she illustrates with the example of how the written word (i.e. documentary sources) is valued more highly than the spoken word (i.e. story-telling). Abigail Masterson talks about the potential of critical theory and discourse analysis as one possibility among others (such as action research) of rectifying the emphasis on 'man-made' language in scientific and other writing.

The recognition that major changes have ocurred in the way that knowledge is produced is apparent in a recent text written by an interdiciplinary group of authors (Gibbons *et al.*, 1994). The authors, from a range of disciplines, including education, sociology, science policy and political science, describe the shift from the conventional, scientific mode of knowledge (i.e. Mode 1) produced in academic institutions to a new mode of knowledge production (i.e. Mode 2). This new mode of knowledge production is described as 'non-linear' in that it does not depend on hypothesis and theory-testing. Mode 2 knowledge values reflexivity, transdisciplinarity and difference, drawing on a range of settings such as factories and hospitals, sources and processes (including information technology) to produce it. It also supports a research agenda which we propose for nursing, which is committed to exploring and legitimating different knowledge forms.

We conclude the first section of our epilogue with a summary of the key themes which have emerged from reviewing the preceding chapters of the book. We suggest that the themes can be used to inform the nursing research agenda as we move in to the millennium. Our assessment of the key themes which need to be considered are:

- the importance of history in shaping the research context and the contribution of previous research findings

- the definition of nursing and nursing research as human endeavours rather than as objects for detached study
- the centrality of reclaiming a passion for caring in nursing and nursing research
- the provision of positive protection (as opposed to negative defences) for nurses to help their engagement in the emotional labour of nursing and nursing research
- the development of rapport and reciprocity between researchers, practitioners and service users/carers
- demystification as the core of reflection and reflexivity which encourages critical and penetrating questioning
- the power differences between nurses and doctors; nurses, service users and lay carers and their implications for research, practice and the subsequent professionalization of nursing
- the need of nurses/nurse researchers for support and supervision in relation to the emotional and ethical dimensions of their work.

We now consider in the second section of our epilogue the application of these themes to nursing research agendas in the twenty-first century.

Into the millennium: new paradigms for nursing research

The key themes which we have just delineated could indicate that a new paradigm is needed for nursing research which incorporates all the themes, irrespective of the topic being studied. But what does it mean to talk about a new paradigm in research? British social scientists Reason and Rowan (1981) used the term in the research context, to posit an alternative to positivism and traditional scientific method. The conventional aim of research is to test theories and establish proof and truth about the world (i.e. Mode 1 knowledge production). Reason and Rowen's new paradigm research meant collaboration, participation and valuing naturalistic experiences rather than setting up controlled experiments in which the researcher is distanced from the subject. The key tenets of the paradigm (adapted from Reason and Rowan, 1981) include the following:

1 The purpose of research is to discover and expose social rigidities and fixed patterns so as to explore the need for and enable change.
2 Closer relationships between researcher and researched and a shared language and praxis are encouraged.
3 Participation in the research brings its own form of knowing.
4 The outcome of research is new knowledge.
5 Knowledge is power, therefore research can never be neutral.

These tenets in a general sense can be seen as echoing central aspects of the themes from the chapters of this book. But should this be our new paradigm? A feminist researcher, Nielsen, writing in 1990, while welcoming Reason and Rowan's efforts to develop alternatives to positivist paradigms and methodologies, was still not convinced that they went far enough to overturn the assumptions on which positivism and scientific method are based. She states: 'they (Reason and Rowan) do not directly answer the lingering question, How do we know what we know? In other words they do not explicitly lead the researcher out of the "either (objectivism)/or (relativism)" dilemma' (p. 26). Nielsen argued the need to seek an alternative worldview (i.e. one that is woman-centred) to either the one which embraces a variety of perspectives and ways of knowing, as in 'relativism', or the other, which seeks to attain absolute truth, as in positivism. By analogy this would mean nursing developing its own methodology: a question we return to later in the chapter.

In relation to the arguments about positivism and conventional science, our own worldview is almost the opposite of establishing one homogenous truth. Rather than seeing 'truth' as the end point of research, we emphasize its processual nature which enhances the researcher's ability to live with the inevitability of uncertainty, and to value difference and diversity. We agree that the emphasis on dualism (mind/body; subjective/objective divide) as an underlying philosophical tenet is problematic. As Betsy Ettore (1980, p. 8) put it: 'Patriarchal thinking confuses women by telling them there is a fundamental dualism in the acquisition of human knowledge. There is "subjective experience" and the "objective interpretation" of it.' The polarization of the subjective and the objective falsifies experience and reality, and the possibility of knowing them. Du Bois (1983) commented that they are not independent of each other, nor should they be, since both are modes of knowing, analysis, interpretation and understanding. The danger in not challenging head on the relativist versus objectivist dichotomy is illustrated by the critique that positivism strips research of its context. Despite the best of intentions, this critque is also valid when applied to the relativist's perspective since:

> Concepts, environments, social interactions are all simplified by methods [i.e. objectivism and relativism] which lift them out of their social context, stripping them of the very complexity which characterises them in the real world. (Parlee quoted in Duelli Klein, 1983)

In other words, a new paradigm, if that is what is required, needs to consider and understand the implications of Plummer's (1983) comment that all perspectives dangle from each person's personal constructs. Views, truths and conceptions of the 'real' world, therefore, can never be wholly ripped away from the people who experience them. We may need to beware here of rejecting all that has been learned through the use of positivist science. Some of the principles which lead to rigour in research may be important. It is possible to present a very partial view (accepting that all views describe only part of the whole anyway) under the guise of research. The integration of subjectivity does not mean that the researcher's view 'rules O.K!'. The challenge for a new paradigm is to integrate the subjective with the objective in a way which moves beyond the futility of the subjectivity/objectivity divide without falling into the dangers highlighted. Dangers to be avoided include context stripping; producing results following the conventional scientific model which simplify the world in order to make it understandable; withdrawing as a researcher into an assumed position of neutrality; and presenting an idiosyncratic perspective as 'the reality'.

Paradox

The importance of the concept of paradox which challenges the boundaries of the subjectivity/objectivity divide, may be important here. The alignment of undisputed boundaries sits uneasily alongside the notion of contradiction which underlies much of our thinking (and which has its own validity). The concept of paradox offers a framework for handling the ambiguity inherent in contradictions and the movement to this new approach may sit uneasily with current thinking at first. Interestingly, it is a concept used by several authors, including Gosia Brykczyńska, Anne Jones and Olwyn Bamford.

Angie Cotter demonstrates how the concept of paradox can be used as a way of handling contradictions by means of a quotation from the *Observer* magazine. Angie began the methodology chapter of her doctoral thesis with the quotation in which a woman with cancer described her experience and in so doing highlighted the importance of paradox in the understanding of reality:

> Mystery, what a mystery this life is. The plants are filling out. The garden out back of our house sprouts one half-inch here, one half-inch there, and I am changing too; cancer plods on from node to node, remarkable and not remarkable at all, like summer itself. Just another growing season after all. Is this resignation? I hope not. I do not intend to give up without a struggle, but more and more I see myself as a thread in a huge and royal tapestry – important to the central design but having an end, a place, a physical destination.
>
> I think of the young daughter in Satyajit Ray's *Pather Panchali*, spinning, whirling in the rain, her hair flying out like a flag the day she died. No one is special, are they, when all is said and done? And of course each one of us is very special, very singular, carrying weight. I matter. I would like to open the window tonight and yell that outside. *I matter*. Or go down and lie next to the plants and whisper it. (Lynch, 1986, p. 30)

Negotiating new research roles

A related challenge which a new paradigm would need to address is to take on board the fact that, once the credibility of the objectivity/subjectivity divide is accepted, the role of the researcher becomes different. And this has one far-reaching consequence. We researchers have to accept that in studying others we also study ourselves. A psychoanalyst and researcher George Devereux (1967) noted that this:

> explains why so many devices are invented to increase detachment and to ensure objectivity, by inhibiting even a creative awareness of one's fellowship with one's subjects, and why so few are devised to promote empathy, even though the only 'methodologically relevant' empathy is that which is rooted in the recognition that both the observer and the observed are human. (p. 71)

He argues that all research is self-relevant and represents more or less indirect introspection. If this is accepted, then it follows that the consciousness and experience of the researcher should be made explicit in the research. When the researcher is seen as instrument (Field and Morse, 1985), the researcher's experience and perspectives become very important. As Stanley and Wise (1983), feminist sociological researchers, have said, research in essence is the narration to an audience of research experiences as these are interpreted by the researcher. The researcher's cultural values, age, ethnic group, gender and sociopolitical situation affects the resultant research.

As Angie explored nurses' personal experiences of severe acute and chronic illness, in her doctoral research, it seemed appropriate to make explicit her own experiences and consciousness. She decided therefore to include a chapter outlining her own experience of illness as an attempt to move her (i.e. the researcher's) consciousness into a more central position. Some critics may see this approach as too easy and self-involved, but in practice Angie found the reverse to be the case. Self-disclosure makes the researcher vulnerable: in one sense, the researcher's self as well as the research is more available for criticism. The attempt to put oneself under the microscope is in itself quite painful and requires a high degree of rigour and discipline. It is interesting that in our book, it has been those chapters which explicitly touched on personal experiences which have been most problematic for the authors.

New paradigms for caring research

In the approach just described and illustrated by Angie's research, the role of the researcher may have much in common with the psychotherapist. We suggest that a closer examination of this phenomenon may elucidate the question whether nursing research needs to develop its own methodology.

The skills required of both the psychotherapist and the nurse researcher involve a complex, albeit relatively little discussed, set of interpersonal skills. Central to the work of each is the necessity to remain open to people, to allow the element of surprise to creep into the equation and to resist the counter-element of needing to maintain and defend a position in an interaction. Both thus aim to put the (service) user at the centre of care.

Ironically, however, the approach of both disciplines has conventionally been very different. Researchers have been hemmed in by the canons of an objectivity which constantly eludes, as if they could put aside their own subjectivity as easily as taking off a cloak. Psychotherapists, however, proceed through knowing their own subjectivity, using themselves as a tool in the therapeutic attempt. This is not unlike Field and Morse's (1985) description of the researcher as instrument, nor Brown and Harris' (1979) claim that the most sensitive measuring instrument is the human brain. Viewing the researcher as a research instrument also addresses Feyer-abend's (1978) criticism of 'the idea of a universal and stable measuring instrument that measures any magnitude, no matter what the circumstances'(p. 98). Conventional science, which Feyerabend views as unrealistic, regards the research instrument (such as the questionnaire or checklist) as the objective tool from which the researcher can disengage. Seeing researchers and not their tools as the instrument addressess issues of subjectivity, consciousness and experience so integral to social research.

One case study from nursing research is illustrative here. Sarah Barnes, a nurse researcher, found herself being used as 'a human sponge' during fieldwork on emotions. Pam Smith was the project director of this study which explored the emotional components of nurse–patient interactions. In-depth interviewing was the cornerstone method. Sarah conducted all the interviews and during the process developed in-depth insights into both emotional and conceptual issues relating to the topic. This necessitated frequent discussions and debriefings throughout the process. Sarah began with research agendas based on those used in Pam's research on emotional labour (Smith, 1992). She made it very clear to the participants, nurses and patients on two orthopaedic wards, that she was interested in the emotional components of care. She soon found that the nature of the research generated a range of emotions in the respondents and in herself.

People felt anxious, angry, sad. One way to reduce their anxiety was to show them the agenda of questions before they began. This might seem to go against the qualitative tradition of keeping the interview informal, flexible and friendly, but Sarah found that this technique worked well for her and the interviewees. At the beginning of the interview, Sarah discussed with the person being interviewed that the content was confidential and primarily for research purposes. If issues arose during interview that required follow-up, Sarah agreed to do this only with the express permission of the interviewee.

In some instances the interview became a therapeutic encounter in its own right. Some patients experienced it as the first opportunity in their long, disabling illness, to recount and reflect on the whole story. Sarah decided that she needed to see a clinical supervisor during her research to help her define the boundaries between nurse as counsellor and nurse as researcher. The supervisor gave valuable support, insights and techniques for conducting and handling the interviews effectively and sensitively. This experience was similar to Angie's exploration in her thesis of nurses' own experiences of severe acute and chronic illness. As a student analytical psychotherapist at the time, she chose to use her training analytical sessions for supervision of the research. Many commonalties are seen here with the discussion of researching sensitive topics and the need for clinical supervision, explored in depth by Trudi James and Dawn Whittaker in Chapter 7.

Some of the debates about the interface between psychotherapy and research centre around the more familiar discussions concerning qualitative and quantitative research and whether the two paradigms should be challenged or reconciled.

For Shapiro (1995), a psychotherapy researcher, the quantitative paradigm, encapsulated by the randomized controlled trial (RCT), fails to address the central goal of psychotherapy research. This goal seeks 'to achieve an understanding of the change mechanisms giving rise to clients' clinical improvement' which 'orthodox research methods' fail to do. Shapiro draws on the literature to demonstrate the inadequacies of 'the drug metaphor' for describing the interaction between therapist and patient/client and oversimplifying the process/outcome distinction. Since a good working relationship between therapist and client is a crucial component of effective psychotherapy, the aim of research is to *include* the placebo effect rather than seeking to eliminate it, as required when designing drug trials. Shapiro makes a 'strong case', therefore, for developing innovative research methods and models which go beyond the RCT to understand change processes. Examples of these innovations include analysing the content and subjective effects of the sessions on clients and describing 'the attainment of insight'.

Should nursing develop its own research methodology?

We now return to a question raised earlier in the chapter about whether nursing should develop a unique methododology. Indeed Thorne (1991) proposed the need for nurse researchers to develop their own qualitative approaches different from those arising from the qualitative paradigm traditionally associated with the disciplines of anthropology, philosophy and sociology. In her view the nursing research enterprise has fundamental differences from the methodologies of phenomenology, ethnography and grounded theory – the three qualitative approaches popular among nurse researchers. She identified the strengths and weaknesses of each approach which she argued, focus on three different levels: the individual (phenomenology); culture (ethnography); and society (grounded theory). Thorne ascribed the popularity of these approaches among nursing researchers to their incorporation in the research process of such notions as empathy and meaning, which are central to the nursing research enterprise.

She encouraged nurse researchers to go beyond the data-collection methods of observation and interviews traditionally associated with qualitative approaches to include clinic and public documents, lay literature and the popular press. Everitt and colleagues (1992), social work practitioners and researchers, also include such sources in their definition of research methods. In Chapter 5, Abigail Masterson shows us how public documents and the press are key to discourse analysis. We will also demonstrate later in this chapter how lay literature, (namely Eva Hoffman's memoirs), can be used to inform and enrich the research enterprise.

Nurses' central role as clinicians and researchers necessarily focuses them on the need for practical research applications rather than purely theoretical ones. Helen Mann in Chapter 8 and Anne Jones and Olwyn Bamford in Chapter 9 demonstrate this focus. In Chapter 6, Gosia Brykczyńska highlights the importance of ethical concerns which impinge on the potential paradox between the nurse's role as carer and researcher. Trudi James and Dawn Whittaker, authors of Chapter 7, show how the interface of the roles can create dilemmas for the practitioner researcher but also create the need for rapport and reciprocity. The centrality of the practitioner role in nursing research, highlights for Thorne the difficulty of maintaining objectivity.

It is possible, therefore, that there are phenomena unique to nursing, which necessitate the development of its own qualitative research approach. It is certainly Thorne's belief that nursing's distinguishing characteristics in relation to its (a) central values (b) capacity for ambiguity (c) complexity and (d) insistence on practical application (1991, p. 191) require nurse researchers to develop their own methodology. Thorne sees nurse researchers as taking a more holistic approach from a focus on either the individual, the cultural or the societal: one which is concerned with the aggregate of human experience for nurses and patients within a unique set of circumstances. In defence of her position, she observed that, in contrast to nurses, educationalists 'have been quite comfortable in adopting and adapting a variety of naturalistic approaches' in order to take research beyond individual and specific contexts (p. 192). In conclusion, Thorne argued that, having agreed there are different ways of 'knowing', there is a need for the emergence of 'a unique process' by which nurses generate their own knowledge.

Can nurse researchers develop a qualitative research approach unique to nursing? Thorne's proposition by which nurse researchers develop a unique research approach is potentially contentious, as the following pros and cons of such an approach indicate.

The pros may include the opportunity to develop applied research knowledge rather than abstract theories about nursing and health care. Furthermore, by developing their own methodologies, nurse researchers may find their voice and give a voice to patients and other nurses. As nurse researchers refine and perfect their own qualitative methodologies, nurse researchers may be able to offer viable alternatives to the dominant quantitative trend within health services research. Again, these proposals are not dissimilar to the key tenets of Reason and Rowan's new paradigm research.

The cons of developing qualitative research approaches unique to nursing, may include a tendency to isolate nursing research from theoretical and methodological developments in other disciplines. Nurse researchers may also lose out on funding opportunities given the current NHS R&D strategy's emphasis on quantitative research. They may also risk narrowing their horizons to concentrate on micro (clinical nursing interventions) rather than incorporating macro (policy) research issues and implications.

The qualitative/quantitative research distinction

In the above discussion about the possibility of new paradigm research in nursing, we have drawn on a number of disciplines to elucidate points. We wish to make it clear that it is our view that nursing does not so much need to develop its own paradigm but instead develop its own perspective and stance. We therefore favour an eclectic approach to nursing research. Similarly, rather than challenging one paradigm over another, nurse researchers Haase and Myers (1988) propose a reconciliation between the two. They write:

> A reconciliation of ideas is often attained by emphasising the similarities or commonalties while weighing the impact of true differences. Efforts to integrate paradigms may be enhanced by the same process. Although there is a difference in purpose between qualitative and quantitative approaches, it is helpful, for comparison, to view this difference as one of emphasis. (p. 130)

The emphasis in quantitative approaches is described as 'confirmation of theory by explaining' in contrast to the qualitative paradigm which 'has emphasized discovery and meaning by describing'. Understanding, therefore, in Haase and Myers' view, becomes 'the orientating factor in reconciling assumptions' underpinning the two paradigms.

Triangulation provides a useful illustration. It is described by these same authors as 'one attempt at recognition of both assumptions and methods' (p. 135) in that it permits the incorporation of multiple theories, methods, researchers and data sources into the research process.

According to Denzin (1989) who popularized the use of triangulation among sociologists, it is not designed to capture an 'objective reality'. Rather, the researcher adopts an interpretive approach by using different methods to give an in-depth understanding of the phenomena under study and a 'negotiated reality' of the research setting. This point is illustrated by the following quotation in which Denzin states:

> Methods are like the kaleidoscope: depending on how they are approached, held, and acted toward, different observations will be revealed. This is not to imply that reality has the shifting qualities of the colored prism, but that it too is an object that moves and that will not permit one interpretation to be stamped upon it. (p. 235)

Another perspective on triangulation can be gained by reading Eva Hoffman's (1989) memoir which describes her North American experience as a Polish Jewish immigrant and the painful transition from one language and culture to another. As an adult in New York's literary society, while at a party, she reflects on the transition. She writes:

> A voice, almost unconscious, keeps performing an inaudible, perpetual triangulation – that process by which ancient Greeks tried to extrapolate, from two points of a triangle drawn in the sand, the moon's distance from the earth . . . I am here, feeling the currents of conflict and warmth, but from that other point in the triangle, there is just one arbitrary version of reality. Nothing here has to be the way it is . . . It's just an awareness that there is another place – another point at the base of the triangle, which renders this place relative, which locates me within that relativity itself. (p. 170)

Hoffman's account is reminiscent of Denzin's description of the kaleidoscope which reminds the reflective researcher that observation of the research setting is a 'negotiated reality' open to a multiplicity of interpretations.

Conclusion

In this final section of the book we wish to reflect on what has gone before and where it may lead. Each author demonstrates how research questions are influenced by who they are, according to their race, class, sexual orientation, gender and personal trajectory. By this we mean our life histories and experience of nursing practice, research and education. The practice-led chapters highlight the central importance of the research and development divide – for what use is research if it is not implemented? There are also pointers in Maureen Lahiff's chapter as to why research may not be implemented. Other authors, such as Gosia Brykczyńska, Anne Jones and Olwyn Bamford, look at refocusing on the synthesis and/or accepting the paradox inherent in caring and nursing research. Colleen Wedderburn Tate, Maureen Lahiff and Maria Lorentzon also describe the trends towards multidisciplinary research, audit and evaluation and the fostering of an evaluative culture, based on medical tenets. A case study of a methodology (discourse analysis) which may lead to liberation and empowerment of nurses, service users and their carers is given. The book highlights the need for support for nurses in their difficult task of making sense of the multiplicity of meanings which research from a practice-based discipline, with an emphasis on caring involves. Clinical supervision may play a key role here.

Another central theme emerging from the book is the importance of research's ability to demystify – to lead us on towards 'a people's science', understandable to the people. It is here that nursing and nursing research may have to decide where it sits in relation to discussions about power relations in health care. There is an acceptance which has been shown throughout the chapters concerning the power relationships persisting between doctors and nurses. However, it is arguable that nursing and nursing research is only just feeling its way towards an acknowledgement that while nurses may not feel themselves as powerful *vis-à-vis* doctors, we nevertheless occupy a privileged position *vis-à-vis* patients/service users and their carers. In short, nurses hold power over patients in the sense that the patient is, in greater or lesser measure, dependent on the nurse for assistance towards their recovery/rehabilitation/maintenance of health.

But what does the book have to offer in terms of new models of research? The key themes drawn from the chapters and listed above show the way. Throughout the book an importance on history, biography and salvaging the subjective is discernible. Further, it indicates that nursing and nursing research need not be afraid of recognizing the importance of much of the work we do, even if this seems like naming the unnameable because it falls under the aegis of emotional labour. Our perspective is not so much that a new paradigm is needed for nursing alone but that nursing and nursing research need to wake up to the contributions which other disciplines bring to the research endeavour of nursing and to the fact that this endeavour is a shared one. Only then can nurses go beyond multidisciplinary endeavours to embrace interdisciplinary ones. Arguably we need a 'people's science' for the millennium and nurses/nurse researchers need to work with others outside nursing, including service users and carers to develop this. Nursing will have its own perspective and stance on theories of research but these will only be meaningful to the wider world if that wider world can relate to them as having a place in the context of the whole tapestry.

Acknowledgements

The authors would like to thank Vicky Franks for her comments on an early draft of this chapter and for her insights into psychotherapy and the research process.

References

Bowles G and Duelli Klein R (eds) (1983) *Theories of Womens' Studies*. Routledge & Kegan Paul, London: 88–104.

Brown G W and Harris T (1979) The sin of subjectivism: a reply to Shapiro. *Behavioural Research and Therapy* 17: 605–13.

Collins H L (1988) When the profit motive threatens patient care. *Registered Nurse* 10(8): 74–83.

Denzin N (1989) Strategies of multiple triangulation. In *The Research Act: A Theoretical Introduction to Sociological Methods*. McGraw Hill, New York: 234–47.

Department of Health (1994) *Supporting Research and Development in the NHS (Culyer Report)*. HMSO, London.

Devereux G (1967) *From Anxiety to Method in the Behavioural Sciences*. Morton and Co, The Hague.

Du Bois B (1983) Passionate scholarship: notes on values, knowledge and method in feminist social science. In Bowles G and Duelli Klein R (eds) *op. cit.*

Elliot E A (1989) The discourse of nursing: a case of silencing. *Nursing and Health Care* 10 (10): 539–43.

Ettore B (1980) Feminist theory: some methodological considerations. Unpublished paper presented at the 1980 BSA conference.

Everitt A, Hardiker P, Littlewood J and Mullender A (1992) *Applied Research for Better Practice*. Macmillan, Basingstoke.

Feyerabend P (1978) *Science in a Free Society*. Verso, London.

Field P A and Morse J (1985) *Nursing Research: The Application of Qualitative Approaches*. Chapman & Hall, London.

Gibbons M, Limoges C, Nowotny H, Schwartzman S, Scott P and Trow M (1994) *The New Production of Knowledge*. Sage, London.

Haase J and Myers S T (1988) Reconciling paradigm assumptions of qualitative and quantitative research. *Western Journal of Nursing Research*. 10(2): 128–37.

Hoffman E (1989) *Lost in Translation: A Life in a New Language*. Penguin Books, Harmondsworth.

Lynch D (1986) Coming to terms with cancer. *Observer* magazine, 16 September: 30–6.

Neuberger J (1993) Why not ask the experts? *Health Services Journal*, 30 September: 21.

Nielsen J (1990) Introduction. In Nielsen J (ed.) *Feminist Research Methods: Exemplary Readings in the Social Sciences*. Westview Press, Boulder.

Parlee M B (1983) quoted in Duelli Klein R, How to do what we want to do: thoughts about feminist methodology. In Bowles G and Duelli Klein R, *op.cit.*

Plummer K (1983) *Documents of Life: An Introduction to the Problems and Literature of the Humanistic Method*. Allen & Unwin, London.

Reason P and Rowan J (1981) *Human Inquiry: A Sourcebook of New Paradigm Research*. John Wiley, Chichester.

Shapiro D (1995) Finding out how psychotherapies help people change. *Psychotherapy Research* 5(1): 1–21.

Smith P (1992) *The Emotional Labour of Nursing: How Nurses Care*. Macmillan, Basingstoke.

Smith P, Towers B, Mackintosh M and Jennings P (1996) The integration of health and social care for the elderly in one local authority. A Consultancy Report, unpublished.

Stanley L and Wise S (1983) *Breaking Out: Feminist Consciousness and Feminist Research*. Routledge & Kegan Paul, London.

Thorne S E (1991) Methodological orthodoxy in qualitative nurisng research: analysis of the issues. *Qualitative Health Research* 1(2): 178–99.

Traynor M and Wade B (1994) *The Morale of Nurses Working in the Community: A Study of Three NHS Trusts: Year 3*. The Daphne Heald Research Unit, Royal College of Nursing, London.

United Kingdom Central Council for Nursing, Midwifery and Health Visiting (1992) *The Scope of Professional Practice*. UKCC, London.

Wade B (1996) *The Changing Face of Community Care for Older People: Whose Choice?* Royal College of Nursing, London.

Wertheim M (1995) *Pythagoras' Trousers: God, Physics and the Gender Wars*. Fourth Estate, London.

Index